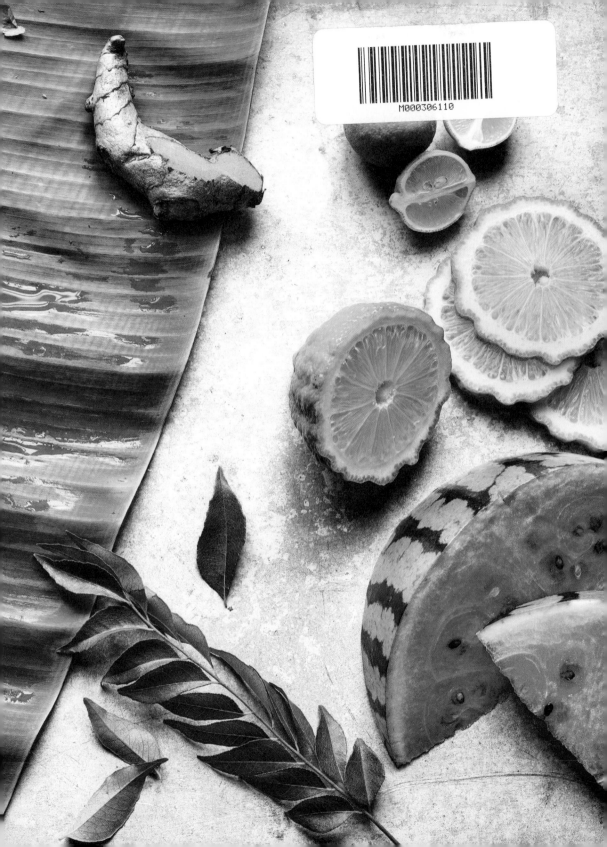

DAN TOOMBS

THE CURRY GUY LIGHT

Over 100 healthy Indian restaurant classics and new dishes to make at home

Photography by Kris Kirkham

Hardie Grant

QUADRILLE

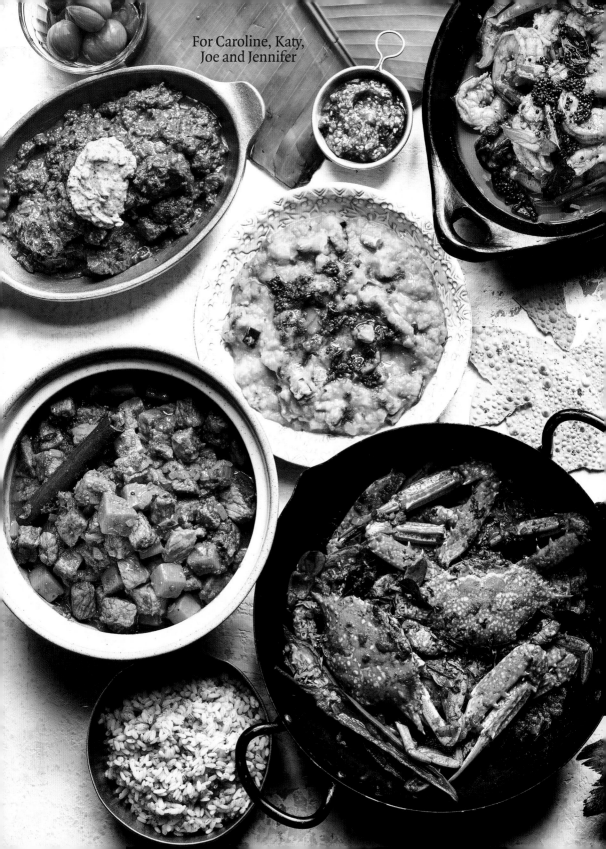

For Caroline, Katy,
Joe and Jennifer

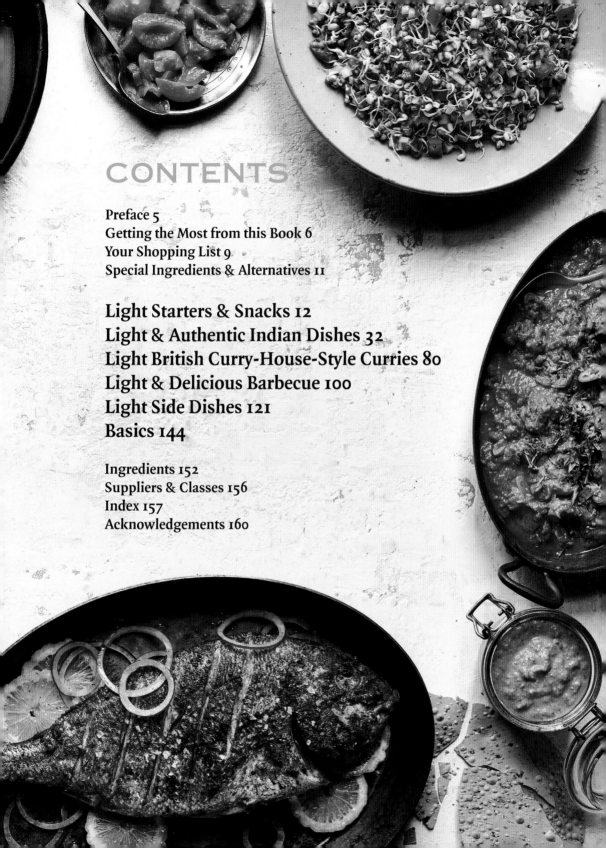

CONTENTS

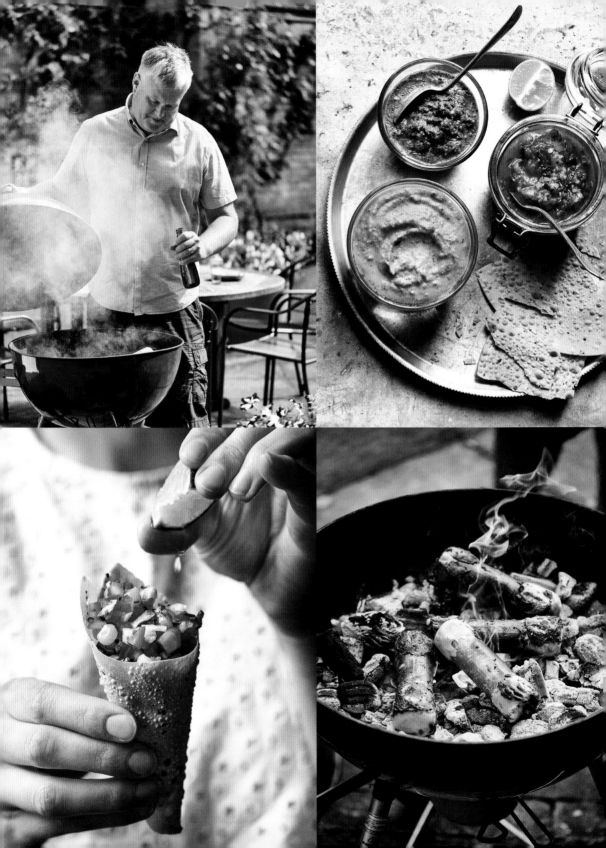

PREFACE

I got the idea for this book after a dinner party my wife and I had for ten friends. We knew that two of them were vegetarian and one was diabetic, so we planned our curry feast so that everyone would find things they could eat. When our guests arrived, we learned that one had starved herself all day because she had recently joined a slimming group and didn't want to miss out on any of the dishes we put on the table. She needn't have done that as we had prepared a Goan meal that was light and in no way calorific.

At that time, I was drafting a book of Goan recipes after a trip there, and this party was our chance to try out some of the recipes on friends. We were amazed that all the food went, as we had made one heck of a lot! That evening, however, I changed my mind about writing the Goan cookbook. What if I could write a cookbook of light recipes that tasted as good as regular versions?

In the following weeks, I managed to convince my wife that we had to go to Kerala in southern Indian to get even more light recipe ideas that were not only good for you but enjoyable to eat, just like the Goan food we loved. We experienced some awesome food over there, and I got to meet and learn from some amazing chefs. This book is greatly down to what I learned while there. These authentic recipes are naturally healthy and easily adapted to most diet plans.

As the book progressed, I decided I didn't want to just feature authentic recipes from the Indian subcontinent, as delicious and light as they were, but also a good selection of British curry-house favourites. This proved quite easy, as cooking with fresh spices means you can use less fat and salt while not compromising on flavour. I had to adapt the cooking methods, but the curries tasted just as good. I started by developing a reduced-fat base curry sauce and then used this to develop lighter versions of the most popular British curry-house-style recipes. I then posted them on my blog for all to try. The response I got was exactly as expected: people were delighted with the lighter versions of their favourite curries that still tasted like those at their local curry house. They wanted and asked for more recipes.

In this book I have set out to produce a selection of recipes that will suit a variety of diets. If you don't feel that fat is a problem, feel free to add more. If white carbs like white rice and naan are what you are trying to avoid, check out the tasty alternatives. All my recipes can be used as templates, and you can adjust them to your preferences or enjoy the alternatives instead.

Authenticity is very important to me, which is why you can make any authentic Indian curry in this book and know you are eating light. In a couple of the British curry-house curries, I reduced the fat and/or sugar content by using excellent substitutes, but if full-fat cream or sugar isn't a problem for you, you can substitute that right back in!

One thing I can assure you is that not one recipe made it into this cookbook that I didn't feel tasted spot on! I even had numerous people do blind taste tests, comparing full-fat versions to low-fat versions, and the recipes all tasted just as good!

I hope you enjoy these healthy recipes. If you have any questions about any of them please get in touch. I manage all my social accounts, so when you ask a question it will be me who answers. I'm @TheCurryGuy on Twitter, Facebook and Instagram, and would love to hear from you. I can also be contacted at dan@thecurryguy.com.

Happy Cooking!

D-28

GETTING THE MOST FROM THIS BOOK

I developed the recipes in this book so that you can enjoy them without any guilt. These aren't 'diet' recipes, but they are naturally lower in calories and fat. The authentic Indian recipes were written exactly as I learned them, though I have recommended substitutes for ingredients that may be difficult to find. I didn't want you not to make a recipe just because you couldn't source fresh curry leaves or kokum! Just make the recipe using my alternative suggestions or omit the ingredient and it will be as good, I promise.

One thing I have enjoyed most about writing my books is the interaction I have had through social media with people who purchased them. I have been asked many recipe questions, some repeatedly. This has made it easier for me to write this book as I have been able to consider the most-asked questions and address them throughout the book. To help you more easily find the recipes you want to try, each recipe has been labelled with one or more badges (such as Gluten free, Vegan, Vegetarian, Make in 30 minutes or less, etc.).

RECIPE LABELS

 30 minutes or less: Look for this when you want to whip something up quickly.

 Fermenting, marinating, resting or soaking time: Just follow the preparation instructions and let nature take its course. I have included this badge so that you know you will need to do a little forward preparation.

 Gluten free (GF): I am always asked which of my recipes are gluten free. Most are. Just look for this badge.

 Vegetarian (V): Look for this badge for vegetarian recipes. Most other recipes can easily be made vegetarian. Substitute veggies, legumes, lentils and/or the veggie kebabs as you see fit.

 Vegan (VE): Most of the recipes can be made vegan but look for this sign for those that are already vegan.

CALORIE & CARB COUNTS

If you are counting your calories and/or carbs, you will find both calorie and carbohydrate counts at the top right of each of the main recipes. For simplicity, I have given counts for the serving size suggested, unless I've specified another quantity, such as per bhaji or tablespoon.

A NOTE ABOUT RECIPE MEASUREMENTS

OIL

In south-Indian cooking, oil is kept to a minimum, and my recipes reflect this. In my BIR (British Indian Restaurant) curries, I have substantially reduced the oil quantities. A typical curry-house curry for one could contain up to 4 tablespoons of oil. That's why you often see a layer of oil at the top of takeaway curries. I have found that a lot less oil can be used without any loss of flavour.

SPICES

Get to know your spices. I have suggested measures for my recipes that suit me, but you can always add less or more to taste. If you don't like spicy curries, add less chilli powder than suggested. You can always add more to taste later, but once a sauce is too spicy it is difficult to cool it down.

I love how in many Indian curries meat is kept to a healthy minimum. It is there as a flavouring for the sauce rather than being 'the dish'. I have done the same in my recipes for meat, poultry and seafood. The amount of these ingredients you put into your sauce is completely up to you, so add more if you wish or cook the recipes just as they are.

BEANS & LEGUMES

All the recipes that call for beans and legumes (such as black beans and chickpeas) were developed so that you can just open a tin (can) and cook. When I cook at home, I usually use dried beans, which I soak and cook beforehand. I like having more control over the finished texture, and it's cheaper too.

For your information, a standard tin of beans weighs 400g (14oz), which reduces to 250g (9oz) when the water is drained. So if you want to use dried chickpeas and a recipe calls for one 400g (14oz) tin of chickpeas, you need to consider the drained weight. Weigh half as many dried chickpeas as the recipe calls for as they will double in weight when soaked. So, for each 400g (14oz) tin of chickpeas (drained weight 250g/9oz), use 125g (4½oz) of dried chickpeas.

USING OIL & COOKING SPRAY

Many diet plans suggest using low-fat cooking spray instead of oil. Although none of my recipes uses a lot of oil, feel free to experiment with cooking spray. I don't suggest it in all my recipes because oil is an excellent transporter of flavour. Spices and fresh aromatic ingredients can be infused into oil and then stirred into the sauce. This simply isn't possible with cooking spray, and I wanted to keep these recipes as close to, if not exactly like, the real thing as possible.

For the recipes in this book, I mainly suggest using rapeseed (canola) oil, even when other oils, such as coconut oil or ghee, are more authentic. Rapeseed oil is lower in saturated fats and has a high smoking point, making it great for cooking Indian food.

You will see below that the calories in oil can quickly add up, which is why I use so little of it. Just remember that if you want to reduce calories, an additional 2 tablespoons of oil adds 240 calories to a curry to serve four but you can use less or try cooking spray. The thing is, oil makes cooking easier. Frying onion in 3 tablespoons of oil is a lot easier than doing the same in just 1 tablespoon. If you find that in using less oil your ingredients are sticking to the pan or burning, reduce the heat. You can cook in far less oil than is usually used with no loss of flavour.

CALORIES AND FAT IN 1 TABLESPOON OF OIL

Rapeseed (canola) oil = 124 calories, 14g fat, of which 1g is 'bad' saturated fat
Olive oil = 119 calories, 14g fat, of which 2g are 'bad' saturated fats
Coconut oil = 117 calories, 14g fat, of which 12g are 'bad' saturated fats
Melted ghee = 135 calories, 15g fat, of which 9g are 'bad' saturated fats
Mustard oil = 124 calories, 14g fat, of which 1.6g are 'bad' saturated fats

Rapeseed (canola) oil is a really healthy oil to use in cooking, and its high smoking point makes it perfect for cooking Indian food. The oils used by the many chefs and home cooks I met were the less healthy but flavourful coconut oil, mustard oil and/or ghee. In some of my recipes I do suggest using these oils, but you can substitute another oil if you prefer. The flavour of the dish might be slightly different, but it will still be delicious.

HIDDEN FATS

I learned a lot while writing this book. I knew that oil obviously increases fat content but I found that other fats, like those in full-fat yoghurt and coconut, have a way of sneaking up on you. I now use 0% fat yoghurt and limit how much coconut milk I use, as even light coconut milk is high in saturated fats.

Of course, when you are following these recipes, you are in control. If you want to use full-fat coconut cream, do it. If, on the other hand, you would like to use less coconut, you can often substitute a little water or stock.

ABOUT THOSE CARBS

Many people want healthier alternatives to white basmati rice, but it plays too big a part in south Indian cuisine to leave it out of the book. A healthier alternative is Keralan red rice, or matta rice (see page 123). It is lower in calories and has health benefits over white rice. Even healthier is brown rice. Both matta and brown rice do take longer to cook. I serve both of these at home and have grown to prefer their flavour and texture over white.

Both white rice and white flours are refined products that have lost valuable nutrients through processing, so using healthier options is a good idea.

Some people choose not to consume rice and/or flour, so I have included tasty alternatives that are very low in carbohydrates, gluten free and make perfect complementary dishes for your Indian meals.

WHICH SWEETENER?

To achieve sweetness in a curry, white refined sugar is usually used. I use small amounts of sugar in some recipes, either in plain white sugar form or alternatives like honey or jaggery, which are really only slightly 'less

bad' sugar. If you are on a low- or no-sugar diet, some artificial sweeteners can be substituted. Not all artificial sweeteners work in cooking though. I have used sucralose and saccharin with good results. Just remember that they are considerably sweeter than sugar and should be added in small amounts.

BATCH COOKING

Batch cooking is an excellent way of ensuring you always have your favourite low-calorie meals on hand. All the recipes in this book freeze well so what are you waiting for? Spending a bit of time in the kitchen cooking up recipes for later might just save you money too! Following are a few tips on this.

CURRIES, STARTERS & TANDOORI

All of the recipes can be frozen and defrosted with brilliant results, however yoghurt and coconut milk do not freeze well so omit any yoghurt or coconut milk and add them to the defrosted and reheated recipes later. With marinated tandoori meats, you will need to cook and then freeze them. Don't freeze raw excess marinade as it won't freeze well.

COOKED RICE

Rice is better frozen than refrigerated, as refrigerated rice can be a bit dry. I use 500ml (2-cup) glass jars with vented lids, which I fill almost to the top with freshly cooked hot rice and then cover. The steam inside will help ensure the rice is moist. Place the rice in the fridge so that it cools quickly (rice should not be consumed if left at room temperature for longer than an hour), then freeze for up to a month. To reheat, microwave from frozen for 2–4 minutes depending on your microwave. Lift the vent to let out hot steam, then serve.

If you don't have the containers, wrap the rice tightly in cling film. I flatten mine for faster cooking. Microwave the rice pack until the cling film comes free, then serve.

YOUR SHOPPING LIST

Indian recipes can be quite daunting to some. There are so many ingredients! The thing is, many of the ingredients are used all the time in varying amounts. In fact, if you pop to your local Asian grocer, you should be able to find what you need for the majority of the recipes in this book. Most of the ingredients can be purchased at supermarkets and online too. One thing I would like to stress is that you shouldn't be put off making a recipe just because you can't source the more unusual ingredients, like black poppy seeds or dried fenugreek leaves (kasoori methi). I included all the ingredients in the recipes for a reason, so get them if you can, but the recipes will still be delicious and healthy if you can't get hold of some.

WHOLE & GROUND SPICES

Whole spices have a much longer shelf life, so try to buy them in this form. By roasting and grinding your own spices, you will not only get all the amazing flavours and aromas, but you will save money too (see pages 147–50 for information on making your own spice blends). Stored correctly in airtight containers in a dark cupboard, whole spices will keep their freshness for many months. Once ground, however, they begin to lose flavour and should be used within 3–6 months. For best results, use them on the day of grinding. We enjoy our food not only through our mouths but also through our noses, so roasting and grinding your own spices will improve the flavour of your dishes.

If you are a really keen cook you might want to stock up on some commonly used ingredients so that you always have them on hand. I grind all my own spices, but you can purchase them ground and still get good results. Having the ingredients listed below in your store cupboard will make things a lot easier if you want to cook a recipe on a whim. You will get the best deals at Asian grocers, and many of the ingredients can still only be found at these grocers or online. If you are an occasional cook, pick the recipe you want to make and buy only the ingredients listed. I always have the following on hand:

COMMONLY USED WHOLE SPICES

Ajwain (carom) seeds
Black peppercorns
Black poppy seeds
Cinnamon sticks
Cloves
Cumin seeds
Dried fenugreek leaves (kasoori methi)
Fennel seeds
Fenugreek seeds
Green cardamom pods
Mace
Mustard seeds
Nutmeg
Sesame seeds
Star anise
Whole dried Kashmiri chillies

COMMONLY USED GROUND SPICES

Remember you can purchase many of these whole and grind them yourself:
Amchoor (dried mango powder)
Asafoetida
Black pepper
Ground coriander
Ground cumin
Ground turmeric
Kashmiri chilli powder (see page 11)
Paprika

Purchase these ready-made or make
your own:
Curry powder
Chaat masala (see page 148)
Garam masala (see page 146)
Tandoori masala (see page 148)

My spice blends are also now available to
purchase online from Spice Kitchen (see the
suppliers on page 156).

FLOURS

Chickpea flour
Coconut flour
Cornflour (cornstarch)
Coarse semolina
Plain (all-purpose) flour
White or brown rice flour

LENTILS & PULSES

Chana dhal
Masoor dhal
Toor dhal
Whole moong (mung) dhal

SWEETENERS

Choose ones that work best for your diet
plan. Artificial sweeteners such as sucralose
and saccharin work in cooking. Otherwise,
if opting for natural sweeteners, go for:
Honey
Jaggery
White sugar

OILS & FATS

Butter (unsalted)
Coconut oil
Ghee
Mustard oil
Rapeseed (canola) oil

SOURING AGENTS

Kokum
Tamarind (block)
Tamarind (concentrate) (see page 149)

RICE

Brown basmati rice
Matta rice (see page 123)
White basmati rice

FRESH INGREDIENTS

Coriander (cilantro)
Curry leaves (don't purchase dried as they
have little flavour)
Garlic
Ginger
Lemongrass
Onions
Tomatoes
Other vegetables as required

TINNED AND BOTTLED INGREDIENTS

Chickpeas
Chopped tomatoes
Light coconut milk
Rapeseed (canola) oil

SPECIAL INGREDIENTS
& ALTERNATIVES

KOKUM & TAMARIND

Many recipes in southern India call for kokum or tamarind. They have a sour and subtly sweet flavour. Kokum is the dried skin from the kokum berry. The blacker the skin, the fresher it is. It isn't used much outside of southern India, but is really good. Kokum is usually used in seafood curries and I love its tangy flavour. It isn't as easy to find as tamarind, but you can purchase it online (see the list of suppliers on page 156).

Tamarind comes both in block form and also as a concentrate. You can make your own tamarind concentrate paste from block tamarind, which is better than any concentrate you can purchase. I explain how to do this on page 149. Shop-bought tamarind concentrate is fine to use though.

Tamarind and kokum can be substituted for each other, but they do taste different. If a recipe calls for 4 dried kokums, you can substitute 4 teaspoons of tamarind paste or concentrate. Likewise, if a recipe calls for 4 teaspoons of tamarind paste or concentrate, you can use 4 pieces of dried kokum skin.

If you are unable to purchase either, add lemon or lime juice to taste, which will give the dish a nice sour flavour, but will not achieve the same beautifully dark colour or the unique flavours.

KASHMIRI CHILLI POWDER

This is a medium-hot chilli powder that is used a lot all over India. Although considered medium-hot by many, some might well find it a bit too spicy. If in doubt, use less than called for in a recipe – you can always add more, but it is difficult to cool a curry down if you add too much. Although I suggest using Kashmiri chilli powder in my recipes, don't fret if you can't source it – instead, use one that you can conveniently purchase.

GARLIC, GINGER & CHILLI PASTES

Garlic paste, ginger paste and a mix of garlic and ginger paste can all be purchased at Asian grocers and many supermarkets. You can buy it in jars and frozen, which is my preference. You can also make it yourself quite easily: simply blend equal amounts of garlic and ginger with a little water until you get a paste-like consistency. It will keep in the fridge for up to three days and can also be frozen. I freeze mine in 2-tablespoon ice-cube trays and then transfer to a freezer bag and defrost when needed. Chilli paste can also be made and stored in the same way. This is really convenient and could also save you money if your chillies are beginning to go off. Just blend them into a paste with a drop of water and use whenever finely chopped chillies are called for in a recipe.

COCONUT

Coconut plays a big part in many of the recipes in this book. I often recommend using fresh or frozen grated coconut. You can substitute dried coconut flakes or desiccated coconut instead – just soak about half the weight called for in water for 30 minutes, then dry off and use as directed in the recipe.

Coconut milk is used in many recipes. You probably know that it is not low in calories! I have substituted light coconut milk, but feel free to use the full-fat version if you prefer.

LIGHT STARTERS & SNACKS

I don't know about you, but when I'm trying to eat
light, my first thought usually isn't 'What can I have
as a starter?' The thing is, eating light doesn't have
to mean giving up on social get-togethers altogether.
I still enjoy having friends and family over for a meal.
In this section you will find some of my favourite light
recipes that are perfect for starting off a meal – or they
could even be served as a light weekday meal on their own.
The portions might be small, but the flavours are strong!
Sometimes I just make two starters and call that dinner.
Who says you can't eat well when you're cutting back?

SWEETCORN CHAAT

SERVES 4

I love a good chaat, and this sweetcorn chaat is simply delicious. Only a small amount of butter is used, but you could actually leave the butter out if you're really cutting back. Me? No way! The fine sev – a deep-fried gram (chickpea) flour crunchy topping that is often added to chaats – can be difficult to find, though it is available online. It can be omitted from this recipe if you like. Although I hope you try the homemade chutney recipes needed for this chaat, they are available ready-made at Asian shops.

PREP TIME: 10 MINS
COOKING TIME: 5 MINS

1 potato, peeled and cut into
    small cubes
1 tsp butter
300g (11oz) tinned (canned)
    sweetcorn, drained
1 tsp red chilli powder
½ tsp garam masala (see page
    146)
½ tsp chaat masala (see page
    148)
1 medium onion, finely chopped
2 medium tomatoes, diced
3 tbsp finely chopped coriander
    (cilantro)
4 tbsp coriander and mint
    chutney (see page 132)
4 tbsp date and tamarind
    chutney (see page 132)
Salt, to taste
3 tbsp fine sev (optional)

Bring a saucepan of water to the boil and cook the potato cubes for 10 minutes, or until soft, then drain. Melt the butter in a frying pan and sauté the sweetcorn and potato for about 1 minute. Add the chilli powder, garam masala and chaat masala and stir well to combine. Transfer to a bowl and allow to cool.

Stir the onion, tomatoes and coriander into the sweetcorn mixture. Drizzle with the chutneys. Season with salt and sprinkle with the fine sev (if using).

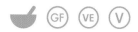

BAKED ONION BHAJIS
MAKES 20

Who doesn't love a good onion bhaji or two when they go out for a curry? Deep-frying them is of course the easier and fattier option, and there is a lot of mess to clean up. I developed this recipe using traditional curry-house techniques to make the perfect batter. The sliced onions are salted to release moisture and to soften them, then the remaining ingredients are mixed in. The resulting bhajis are crisp, healthy and delicious! You can eat two (and perhaps a couple more) without feeling any guilt!

PREP TIME: 10 MINS, PLUS
SITTING TIME
COOKING TIME: 35–45
MINS

3 large onions (about 600g/
    1lb 5oz)
1 tsp fine sea salt
1 tsp cumin seeds
2.5cm (1-inch) piece of ginger,
    peeled and julienned
¼ tsp ground turmeric
¾ tsp ground coriander
3 tbsp finely chopped coriander
    (cilantro)
2 green bird's eye chillies, finely
    chopped
¼ tsp Kashmiri chilli powder
100g (¾ cup) chickpea flour
1½ tbsp rapeseed (canola) oil
Chutney or raita of your choice,
    to serve

Peel and finely slice the onions. Cut each slice into 3cm (1¼-inch) pieces. Place the onions in a bowl and sprinkle with the salt, mixing very well with your hands. Allow to sit for at least 30 minutes or up to 3 hours. When ready to form the bhajis, squeeze the onions with your hands to release the water into the bowl. Add the remaining ingredients up to and including the chilli powder to the bowl and give everything a good stir.

Now sift the chickpea flour over the onion mixture and mix well. There should be enough water released from the salted onions to form a batter that sticks the onions together like you would expect a bhaji to stick together. If too dry, you could add a drop of water, but I have never found this to be necessary. If you add too much water, just sift in a little more flour. Mix in the oil with your hands so that the onions are evenly coated with the oil.

Preheat the oven to 200°C (400°F/Gas 6). Place a sheet of parchment paper on a baking tray (do not use foil as the bhajis will stick to it). Using a spoon or your hands, make 20 equal-sized onion balls and place them on the parchment paper. Bake for about 40 minutes, or until nicely browned. Remember, ovens vary, so check the bhajis from time to time. Serve with a good chutney and/or raita.

NOTE

If you would rather deep-fry the bhajis for up to 27 extra calories per bhaji, heat 10cm (4 inches) of rapeseed (canola) oil to 165°C/330°F in a wok or saucepan and fry them for about 2 minutes until just turning brown. The bhajis will probably still be a bit raw in the middle. Remove from the oil and heat the oil to 185°C/365°F, then fry again for about 2 more minutes until crispy and brown and completely cooked through. You will need to do this in batches. Transfer to paper towels to soak up any excess oil.

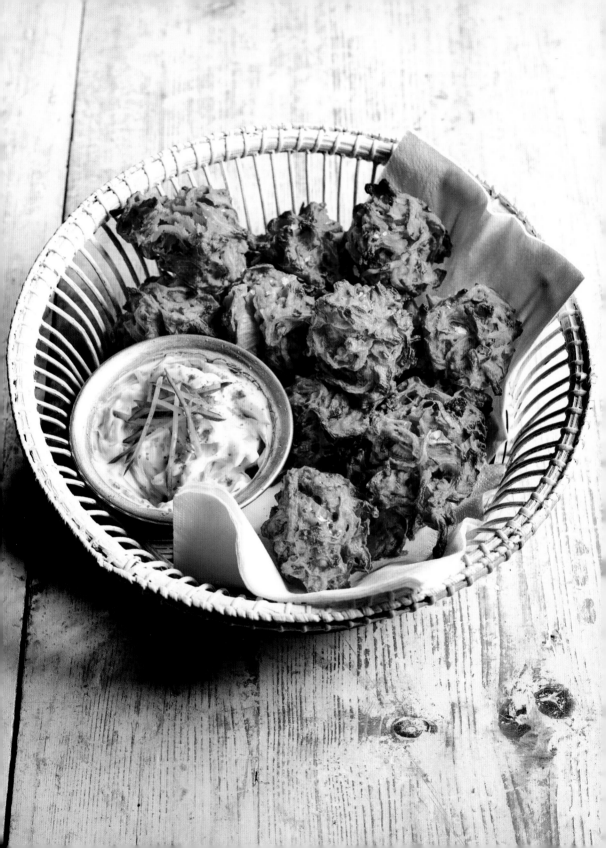

STUFFED PAPAD CONES

MAKES 8

Papad cones make delicious and colourful starters. I learned to make them at a hotel I was staying at in Munnar. I actually thought the cones had been fried, as they were crispy and good. What a great find! When I teach my curry classes, I usually include this recipe. They are fun to make and quite easy too. You can vary this recipe with many different fillings, but the tomato chutney used here is a great place to start. I like to use papads flavoured with cumin and black pepper. These are available at most Asian markets, but you could also use plain ones. No oil is used in this recipe, so you can enjoy these as a quick and healthy snack anytime.

PREP TIME: 10 MINS
COOKING TIME: 15 MINS

3 medium tomatoes
½ onion, finely chopped
2 green chillies, finely chopped
   (more or less, to taste)
3 tbsp cooked sweetcorn
   (colourful but optional)
1 tbsp finely chopped coriander
   (cilantro)
½–1 tsp chaat masala (optional)
   (see page 148)
Salt, to taste
Juice of 1 lime
4 papads, cut in half with
   scissors or a sharp knife

Quarter the tomatoes and remove the seeds so that you are left with tomato petals with most of the excess juice removed. Dice finely and place in a bowl with the remaining ingredients up to and including the lime juice and mix well. Remember that chaat masala (if using) has black salt in it, so this should be considered when seasoning with salt. Place the chutney in the fridge while you make the papad cones.

Heat a dry frying pan over a medium heat and place one of the papad halves in it. Cook for about 15 seconds until it begins to cook through. Use a clean tea (dish) towel to press it down so that it cooks evenly. Flip it over and cook the other side. Repeat by turning again and again until the papad is cooked through and small bubbles appear.

The cut side of the papad will become the top of the cone. While the papad is still hot, roll it into a cone shape and hold the seam for a few seconds until it stays in a cone shape of its own accord. Repeat with the remaining papads.

To serve, fill each cone with the prepared tomato chutney and serve immediately.

NOTE

Once filled with the tomato chutney, the papad cones will become soggy if left too long. So if not serving immediately, fill them just before you want to serve them or let people fill their own cones. The cooked cones can be made a day earlier and stored in an air-tight container.

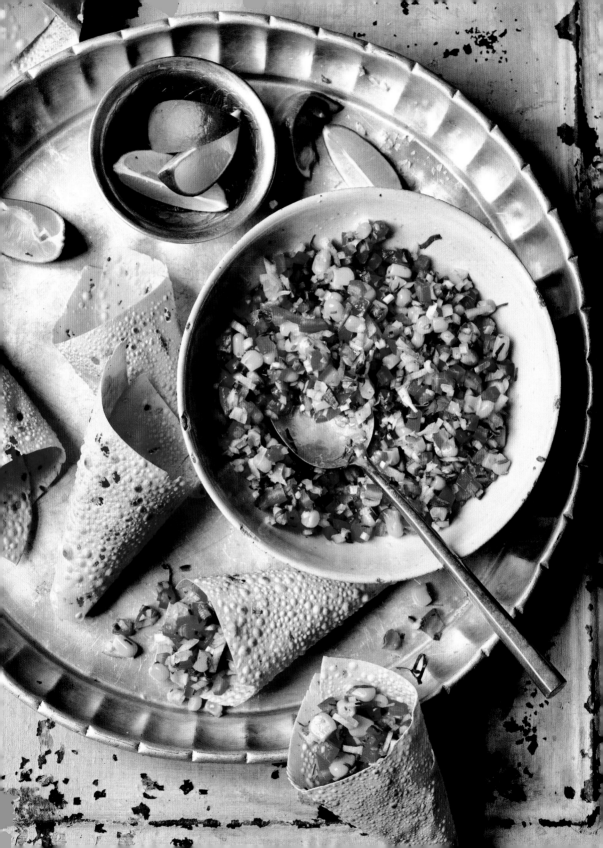

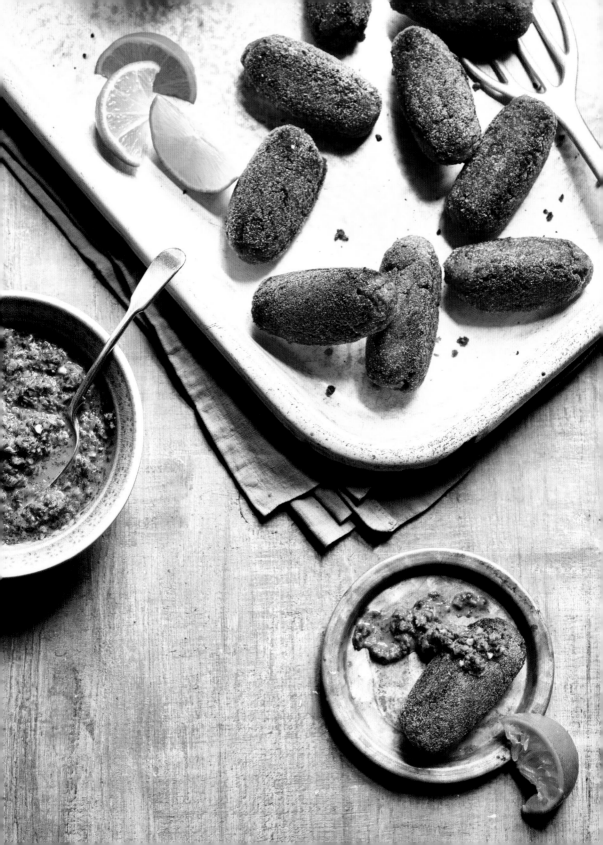

BEEF CROQUETTES

MAKES 12 (SERVES 4 AS A STARTER OR SNACK)

These croquettes are so fall-apart-tender you could eat them without teeth! The meat is cooked before forming it into croquettes, so all you need to do is heat them up and brown them in a pan. A good non-stick pan is not essential but will make cooking with cooking spray easier. Croquettes are usually pan fried, but you can bake them if you prefer, which requires less attention. They are delicious served simply with lime wedges and the coriander and mint chutney on page 132 or a hot sauce of your choice.

PREP TIME: 15 MINS
COOKING TIME: 25 MINS

Cooking spray, as required
1 medium onion, finely chopped
1–3 green bird's eye chillies,
   finely chopped
1 medium tomato, diced
1 tbsp garlic and ginger paste
500g (1lb 2oz) lean beef mince
   (ground beef)
1 tsp ground black pepper
$\frac{1}{2}$ tsp ground turmeric
$\frac{1}{2}$ tbsp garam masala (see page
   146)
$\frac{1}{2}$ tsp chilli powder
$\frac{1}{2}$ tsp salt
1 egg, beaten
10g ($\frac{1}{4}$oz) chopped coriander
   (cilantro)
25g ($\frac{1}{4}$ cup) wholewheat
   breadcrumbs
1 tbsp rapeseed (canola) oil or
   cooking spray
85g ($\frac{1}{2}$ cup) coarse semolina
Flaky sea salt, to taste

Spray a frying pan – preferably non-stick – with cooking spray and place over a medium heat. Fry the onion for 2 minutes, then stir in the chillies, tomato, and garlic and ginger paste. Mix well and add the beef. Stir in the spices so that the meat is nicely coated. Cover the pan and cook for about 10 minutes, or until completely cooked through, then uncover the pan and continue cooking until all the moisture has evaporated; the meat needs to be quite dry.

Allow the meat to cool and then stir in the salt, egg and coriander. Using a food processor, blend the meat to a very smooth paste. Mix in the breadcrumbs using your hands.

Take a piece of meat paste slightly larger than a golf ball and form it into a fat sausage shape. Repeat to form 12 croquettes. The croquettes can be kept covered in the fridge for up to three days until you are ready to fry them.

When ready to cook, spray a non-stick frying pan with cooking spray or use 1 tablespoon of rapeseed oil. Oil will give a crispier exterior and makes cooking less fussy, but both methods work well. Roll the croquettes in the semolina so that they are coated all over. Place the pan over a medium heat and cook the croquettes for about 5 minutes until browned, being sure to roll them around in the pan so that they cook evenly. Season with salt and serve.

Oven method: Preheat the oven to 220°C (425°F/Gas 7). Lightly spray a baking tray with cooking spray. Place the croquettes on the tray and spray them lightly with cooking spray too. Bake for about 20 minutes, or until the croquettes are nicely browned.

STEAMED CHICKEN MOMOS
MAKES ABOUT 24 (SERVES 6)

In my other books, I featured a few popular samosa recipes. I think of momos as a healthier, steamed alternative that are just as good as any samosa I've had! In fact, I prefer them and they are easier and a lot less messy to make. This is a recipe that was sent to me by my friend Santosh Shah, Executive Chef of Baluchi in London. His creative cooking style is amazing, so I'm positive you are going to love this recipe. This dish is delicious served with a simple soy sauce, but I like to serve it with Santosh's roasted tomato and sesame chutney (see page 134). In the photograph opposite, we actually used a slightly different version of this chutney, using half the amount of sesame seeds and blending in a food processor to create a rougher paste. Both of these chutney options are delicious.

PREP TIME: 1 HOUR, PLUS
RESTING TIME
COOKING TIME: 10–12
MINS

FOR THE WRAPPERS
200g (1½ cups) plain (all-
    purpose) flour, plus extra
    for dusting
¼ tsp baking powder
Good pinch of salt
100ml (scant ½ cup) water
3 tbsp cornflour (cornstarch),
    for dusting

FOR THE FILLING
500g (1lb 2oz) raw chicken
    breast, finely chopped (it
    shouldn't look minced, but
    pretty close to that)
1 red onion, finely chopped
2 garlic cloves, finely chopped
5cm (2-inch) piece of ginger,
    peeled and finely chopped
4 green chillies, finely chopped
2 spring onions (scallions),
    chopped
1 tsp black peppercorns, crushed
2 tbsp chopped coriander
    (cilantro)
1 stick of lemongrass, finely
    chopped
50g (1¾oz) butter
1¼ tsp salt
Juice of 1 lemon

Start by making the wrappers. Sieve the flour and baking powder onto a clean work surface. Make a well in the middle and sprinkle in the salt. Add half the water and mix well with your hands. Add the rest of the water and continue to work until the dough is smooth. Knead well for about 5 minutes, then place the dough ball in the bowl, cover and set aside for 30 minutes.

Transfer the dough onto a clean work surface lightly dusted with flour. Roll the dough out with your hands into a long cylindrical shape about 2.5cm (1 inch) in diameter. Cut into 24 or so 2.5cm (1-inch) pieces. Dust with flour and flatten each piece into a circular shape with your hands. Using a rolling pin, roll out each piece into a circle 7.5–9cm (3–3½ inches) in diameter and 2mm thick. Dust the circles with the cornflour (cornstarch) and stack them on top of each other. Cover the wrappers with a damp tea (dish) towel to prevent them from drying out.

To make the filling, mix the chicken with all the other ingredients. When ready to make the momos, take a wrapper, wet the inside circular edge with water, place a heaped teaspoonful of mixture in the middle and fold it over. Press the two corners together to begin the seal. Make small folds towards one of the corners and continue until you have completely sealed the momo, as photographed. This looks great but if you find this difficult, the most important thing is that the momos are sealed shut. They will still taste great! Repeat with the remaining momos.

Transfer the momos to a steamer set at a high heat (you may have to do this in batches) and steam for 10–12 minutes until the filling is cooked through.

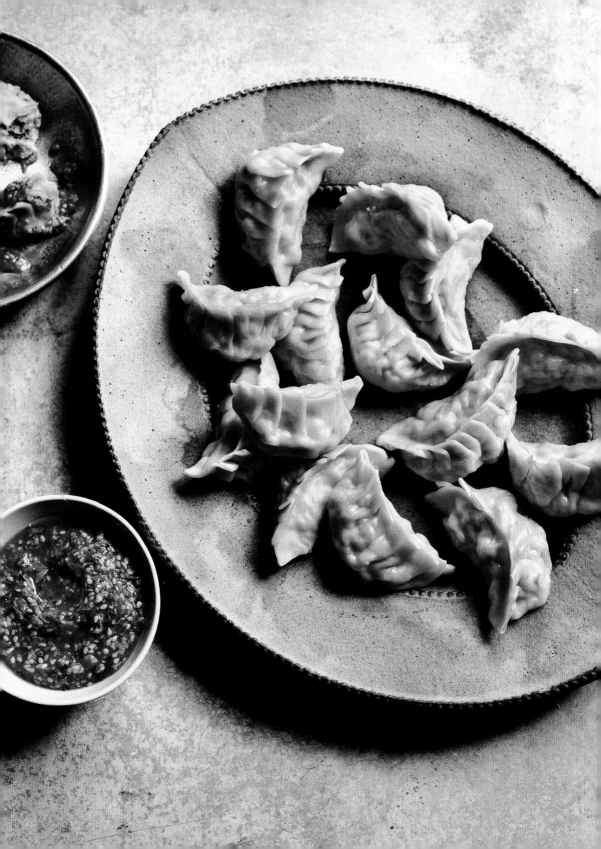

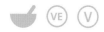

VEGETABLE MOMOS
MAKES ABOUT 24 (SERVES 6)

If you are looking for a meat-free option for the momos on page 20, look no further. I learned to make momos using this filling. The ingredients for this are cheaper too so it is a good one to practise those momo-wrapping skills. One thing I would like to stress is that you shouldn't worry too much about making perfectly folded momos at first. You'll get there with practice, but the most important thing is that the filling is completely sealed inside the wrapper. Pretty or not, they taste great!

PREP TIME: 1 HOUR, PLUS RESTING TIME
COOKING TIME: 10–12 MINS

FOR THE WRAPPERS
200g (1½ cups) plain (all-purpose) flour, plus extra for dusting
¼ tsp baking powder
Good pinch of salt
100ml (scant ½ cup) water
Cornflour (cornstarch), for dusting

FOR THE FILLING
1 carrot, finely diced
1 celery stick, finely diced
5 garlic cloves, finely chopped
2cm (¾-inch) piece of ginger, peeled and finely chopped
½ onion, finely chopped
3 spring onions (scallions), finely chopped
3 tbsp chopped coriander (cilantro)
1 green chilli, finely chopped
225g (8oz) green cabbage, finely sliced and chopped
1 tbsp rapeseed (canola) oil
1 tsp ground cumin
1 tbsp light soy sauce
Salt and freshly ground black pepper, to taste

TO SERVE
Soy sauce or chilli sauce

Start by making the wrappers. Sieve the flour and baking powder onto a clean work surface. Make a well in the middle and sprinkle in the salt. Add half the water and mix well with your hands. Add the rest of the water and continue to work until the dough is smooth. Knead well for about 5 minutes, then place the dough ball in the bowl, cover and set aside for 30 minutes.

Transfer the dough onto a clean work surface lightly dusted with flour. Roll the dough out with your hands into a long cylindrical shape about 2.5cm (1 inch) in diameter. Cut into 24 or so 2.5cm (1-inch) pieces. Dust with flour and flatten each piece into a circular shape with your hands. Using a rolling pin, roll out each piece into a circle 7.5–9cm (3–3½ inches) in diameter and 2mm thick. Dust the circles with the cornflour (cornstarch) and stack them on top of each other. Cover the wrappers with a damp tea (dish) towel to prevent them from drying out.

To make the filling, place all the ingredients into a large bowl and mix well.

When ready to make the momos, take a wrapper, wet the inside circular edge with water, place a heaped teaspoonful of filling mixture in the middle and fold it over. Press the two corners together to begin the seal. Make small folds towards one of the corners and continue until you have completely sealed the momo (as photographed on page 21). This looks great but if you find this difficult, the most important thing is that the momos are sealed shut. They will still taste great! Repeat with the remaining momos.

Transfer the momos to a steamer set at a high heat (you may have to do this in batches) and steam for 10–12 minutes until the filling is cooked through.

Eat immediately dipped in soy sauce and/or chilli sauce.

BAKED GHUGRA
MAKES 20

Ghugra are very similar to samosas and are usually deep fried. This baked version reminds me a lot of Spanish empanadas, but with a lot less fat. The simple filling is packed with flavour, so you aren't going to miss the fat anyway. If working ahead of time, you can make the ghugra and then freeze them. Just take them out and defrost before baking.

PREP TIME: 15 MINS, PLUS
RESTING TIME
COOKING TIME: 35 MINS

250g (scant 2 cups) plain (all-purpose) flour, plus extra for dusting
2 tbsp melted ghee
½ tsp salt
About 250ml (1 cup) water
2 tsp rapeseed (canola) oil
1 tsp cumin seeds
1 tsp sesame seeds
2 green chillies, minced
¼ tsp asafoetida
1 tbsp garlic and ginger paste
225g (1½ cups) frozen peas, roughly crushed
3 tbsp fresh or frozen grated coconut
3 tbsp finely chopped coriander (cilantro)
Juice of 1 lemon
Salt, to taste
1 egg, whisked
Cooking spray, for greasing

Place the flour, ghee and salt in a large mixing bowl. Slowly add the water until you have a firm, workable dough that is only slightly sticky to the touch. Knead directly in the bowl for about 5 minutes, then place a wet tea (dish) towel over the bowl and let the dough sit for at least 30 minutes or overnight.

When ready to cook, heat the oil in a large frying pan over a medium–high heat. When visibly hot, add the cumin seeds, sesame seeds, chillies and asafoetida. Allow to infuse into the oil for about 15 seconds, then add the garlic and ginger paste and fry for a further 30 seconds. Now stir in the peas, coconut and coriander. Reduce the temperature to low, add 3 tablespoons of water, cover and cook for another 5 minutes, stirring regularly, until the peas are soft and the water has evaporated. Squeeze in the lemon juice and season with salt. Transfer to a bowl to cool.

To make the wrappers, divide the dough into 20 equal pieces. Lightly flour a clean work surface and roll each piece into a 7.5cm (3-inch) circle. Place about 1 tablespoon of the pea mixture on each, then fold over into a half-circle. Using a fork, press down on the open seam to close the ghugra.

Preheat the oven to 200°C (400°F/Gas 6). Lightly brush each ghugra with the egg wash and place on a lightly greased baking tray – cooking spray is perfect for this. Place the tray on the middle rack in the oven and bake for 15 minutes. Turn the ghugra over and lightly brush the other side with the egg wash, then return to the oven for a further 10–15 minutes until lightly browned and heated through. Serve hot.

SPICY HOT CHICKEN WINGS
SERVES 4

Did you know that half the calories in chicken wings is in the skin? In Indian cooking, chicken skin is usually removed. It just isn't needed for flavour when the chicken is served with a delicious and spicy sauce. You could either skin the wings yourself or visit your local Asian shop where the butchers do it for you. That's what I do. This recipe was given to me by my friend and chef Moh Hoque, who developed it for a spicy food-eating contest. The Carolina reaper chilli powder is about as hot as it comes, but you could substitute a milder chilli powder or even paprika. In this recipe, the chicken is cooked from raw in the sauce. Another option would be to barbecue the chicken. Try using the marinade from the tandoori chicken tikka on page 102 and marinate for 30 minutes or overnight before grilling it. Then just follow the rest of the recipe. These are delicious served with excess sauce (I often make more), or if you want to cool them down, serve them with a good raita like the cucumber raita on page 136 or the onion raita on page 139.

PREP TIME: 10 MINS
COOKING TIME: 10 MINS

1 tbsp rapeseed (canola) oil
1 tbsp garlic and ginger paste
½ tbsp mixed powder or curry powder
½ tbsp garam masala (see page 146)
1 tsp Carolina chilli powder (more or less, to taste)
1 tbsp tomato purée (see page 146)
1 tbsp sugar or honey
100ml (scant ½ cup) base curry sauce (see page 83)
12 chicken wings, skinned
Juice of 1 lime
Pinch of dried fenugreek leaves (kasoori methi)
Salt, to taste
1 tbsp finely chopped coriander (cilantro)

Heat the oil in a frying pan over a medium–high heat until really hot. Add the garlic and ginger paste and fry for 30 seconds.

Stir in the mixed powder, garam masala, chilli powder, tomato purée and sugar or honey. Give it all a good stir, then stir in the base sauce and bring to the boil. Reduce the heat a little, add the chicken wings and allow them to cook in the simmering sauce for about 7 minutes or until cooked through. If you need to add a little more base sauce or water to cook the chicken through, do it.

To finish, squeeze the lime juice over the top and sprinkle with the dried fenugreek leaves (kasoori methi). Check for seasoning. Sprinkle with the coriander and serve.

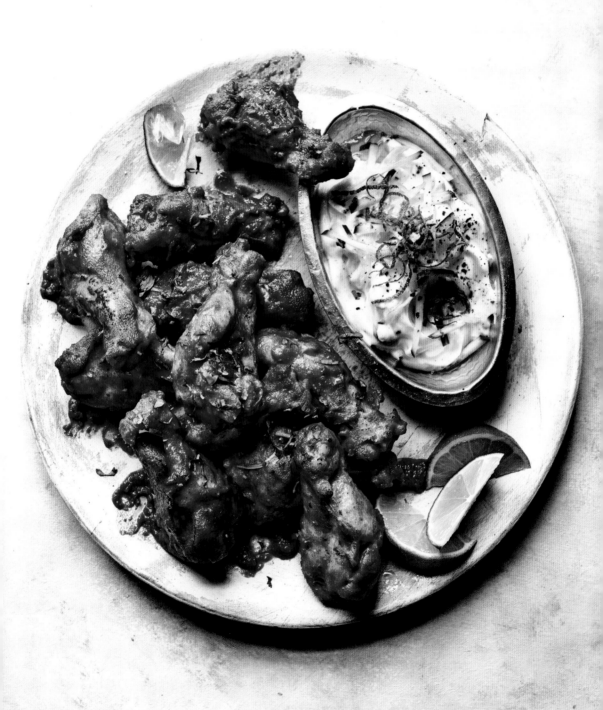

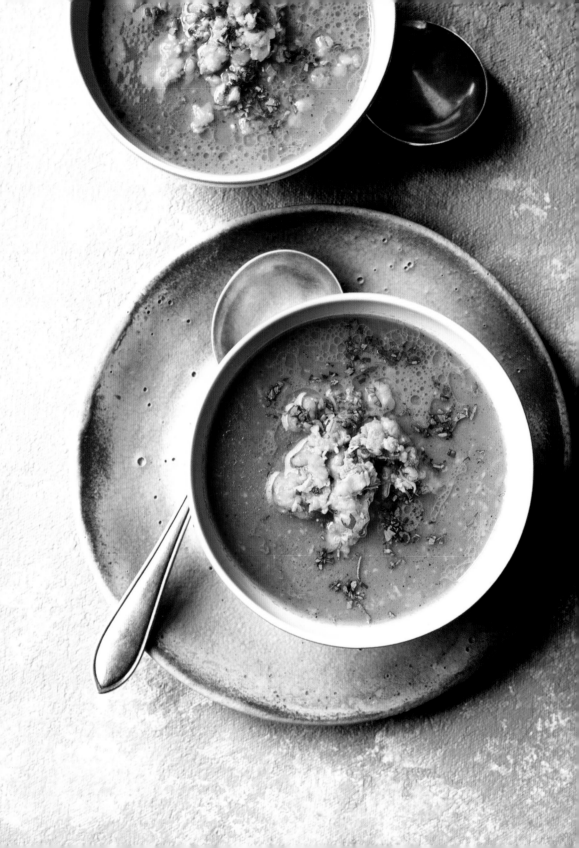

SEAFOOD THENGA PAAL SOUP

SERVES 2

If you want to impress someone with your cooking, this recipe will do it. On a trip to Kochi (Cochin) in Kerala, my wife and I were invited to one of the most amazing meals at Trilogi, in the Crowne Plaza, Kochi. The food was both visually exciting and delicious. This seafood soup was the starter course and I just had to get the recipe! The soup we tried was creamier, which can be achieved by adding a couple of tablespoons of single cream or full-fat coconut milk, but I find this low-calorie version equally delicious.

PREP TIME: 15 MINS
COOKING TIME: 45 MINS

500g (1lb 2oz) fish bones from non-oily fish such as bream, bass or halibut

3 garlic cloves, thinly sliced

2.5cm (1-inch) piece of ginger, peeled and julienned

1 medium onion, sliced

10 fresh or frozen curry leaves

1 tomato, sliced

2 tbsp rapeseed (canola) oil or coconut oil

150g (5½oz) minced seafood (choose a good selection of meaty fish, such as prawns, cod and halibut)

1 tsp asafoetida*

½ tsp ground turmeric

10g (¼oz) tender fresh coconut, cut into small cubes (optional)

80ml (⅓ cup) light coconut milk

Salt, to taste

Juice of ½ lemon

1½ tbsp tamarind paste (see page 149) or concentrate (more or less, to taste)

1 tsp freshly ground black pepper

2 tbsp finely chopped coriander (cilantro)

Place the fish bones in a large saucepan and add the garlic, ginger, onion, curry leaves and tomato. Cover with 2 litres (8 cups) of water and bring to a boil. Reduce the heat and simmer for 30–40 minutes until the water has reduced to about ½ litre (2 cups). Strain the fish stock through a fine-mesh sieve and set aside.

In a separate saucepan, heat the oil over a medium–high heat and stir in the seafood. Add the asafoetida and turmeric and give it all a good stir to combine, then add the reduced fish stock. Bring back to the boil, then add the coconut (if using). Reduce the heat so that the soup is just simmering, then stir in the coconut milk. Season with salt and add the lemon juice. Stir in tamarind paste or concentrate and black pepper. To serve, pour into two warmed bowls and sprinkle with the coriander.

NOTE

*Asafoetida is a much-used spice and flavour enhancer in Indian cuisine. If you are gluten-free, please check the asafoetida packaging as some brands contain wheat flour.

ALLEPPEY SALAD

SERVES 4

This is a recipe I almost didn't include because it's so mind-numbingly easy. It's served at restaurants all over Alleppey and Cochin, and I think it's the perfect healthy way to start a meal. There may not be much to it, but its simplicity made me love the idea of it. Sometimes it's just nice to have a healthy snack before the flavoursome curries are brought to the table. You can see a photo of how I plated this on page 138. It is essential that your veggies are super-fresh and crisp.

PREP TIME: 10 MINS

1 cucumber
2 carrots, peeled if you want
2 medium red onions, finely sliced
2 medium tomatoes, finely sliced
4 green bird's eye chillies, left whole
Juice of 2 limes
Salt and freshly ground black pepper, to taste

Cut the cucumber and carrots at a slight angle into 3mm (⅛-inch) slices. To plate, lay all the vegetables in colourful rows or rounds, as they do in Kerala, or go for a more haphazard look, as I normally do. Top with the chillies and lime juice. Season with salt and black pepper.

STIR-FRIED RECHEADO OKRA

SERVES 4

This is good for the recheado masala paste on page 147. Once you have that made – and I should add that recheado sauce is amazing cooked with vegetables, meat and seafood – you can make this dish quickly and easily. Many people don't like okra because when prepared incorrectly it can become slimy. There are a couple of things you can do to rectify this problem. The one I do most often is to soak the whole okra in vinegar for 30 minutes before rinsing and drying it. Then I slit and fill it. You can also freeze okra before slitting and filling. Once slit or cut, however, it needs to be cooked right away.

PREP TIME: 10 MINS
COOKING TIME: 10 MINS

20 okra, ends trimmed
250ml (1 cup) recheado masala paste (see page 147)
1 tbsp rapeseed (canola) oil

Make a slit down the middle of each okra, leaving the ends uncut. Fill each okra with the recheado masala paste.

When ready to cook, heat the oil in a frying pan over a medium–high heat and fry the okra on all sides for about 5 minutes, or until soft and cooked through. Serve hot.

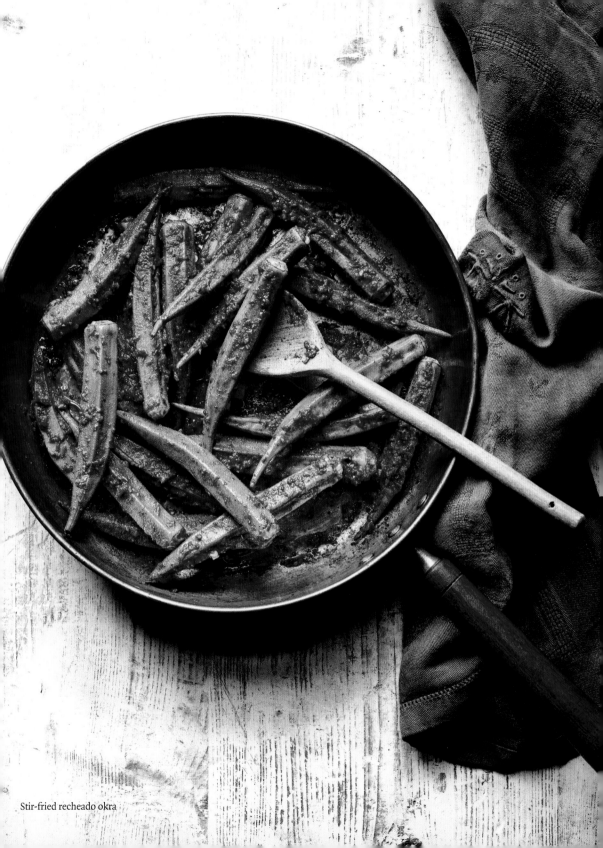

Stir-fried recheado okra

SQUID ROAST
SERVES 6

My wife and I first came across this dish by accident in Alleppey. Kerala's alcohol laws are very strict and we were finding it hard to find a drink – we were on holiday after all! We were told to try a toddy bar up the road from where we were staying. Toddy shacks are all over the place and can be a bit off-putting as you will often see drunk men asleep on the benches after having necked back a bit too much of the cheap, but condoned, palm sap alcohol. Some toddy shacks serve fantastic food too, like the one we first experienced and where we tried their famous squid roast. The toddy was pretty good too. Many chefs just quick-fry the squid in oil, but by cooking it first in water, it becomes very tender and less oil is required for the final cooking. By the way, if you find yourself in Kerala and want to try some toddy and possibly some great local food, look for this sign കള്ള് as they are not always sign-posted in English.

PREP TIME: 10 MINS, PLUS
MARINATING TIME
COOKING TIME: 40 MINS

900g (2lb) squid, cut into 7mm
(¼-inch) rings

FOR THE MARINADE
1 tsp rapeseed (canola) oil
½ tsp salt
1 tbsp garlic and ginger paste
3 green chillies, smashed or
    blended into a paste
2 kokums or 1 tsp tamarind
    paste (see page 149) or
    concentrate
10 fresh or frozen curry leaves
1 tsp ground turmeric

FOR THE MASALA
2 tbsp rapeseed (canola) oil or
    coconut oil
1 tsp black mustard seeds
20 fresh or frozen curry leaves
2 medium red onions, thinly
    sliced
2 tbsp garlic and ginger paste
2 green chillies, finely chopped
1 tbsp chilli powder (more or
    less, to taste)
1 tbsp ground coriander
½ tsp freshly ground black
    pepper
½ tsp garam masala (preferably
    homemade; see page 146)
Salt, to taste

Wash and dry the squid well. Place the squid rings in a large mixing bowl. If you want to include the squid tentacles, go for it. Mix in the oil and salt, then add the remaining marinade ingredients so that the squid rings are nicely coated. Marinate in the fridge for about 1 hour.

Transfer the marinated squid with all the marinade to a saucepan and add about 250ml (1 cup) of water. Bring to a boil, then simmer for 30 minutes until all the water has evaporated. You can add a drop more water during cooking if needed.

Meanwhile, make the masala. Heat the oil in a frying pan over a medium–high heat. Stir in the black mustard seeds and when they begin to pop (after about 30 seconds), add the curry leaves and onions and fry for about 5 minutes until the onions are really soft and translucent. Add the garlic and ginger paste and the green chillies, followed by the chilli powder and ground coriander and fry for about 3 minutes until you have a rather dry, soft onion mixture.

Now stir in the squid with all the ingredients from the pan and sauté well. To finish, stir in the black pepper and garam masala and season with salt.

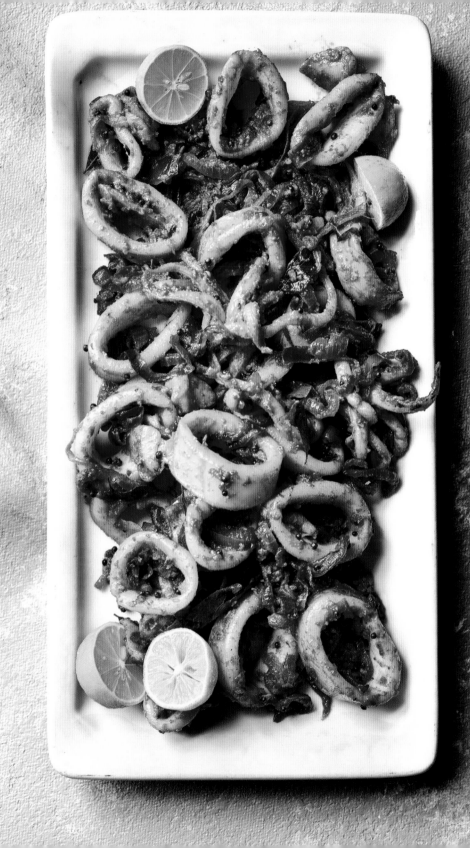

LIGHT & AUTHENTIC INDIAN DISHES

With the exception of a couple of these recipes, you will be making them exactly as I have made them and watched them being made many times. You may be cooking light, but these curries are, and always have been, low-calorie dishes that rely on the quality of the ingredients used and in how the spices are prepared for their amazing flavour. You won't miss the fat because it just isn't needed!

For those recipes where I have made slight reductions in fat, you won't notice the difference there either. Think about the last time you made a good chicken stock or stew – the oil that rises to the top doesn't taste of much. Many people stir that fat back in or skim it off. With the cooking methods used in these recipes, you may need to watch things closely at the beginning, but you will save yourself all that fat at the end. These light recipes take about the same amount of time to make as those using traditional full-fat methods, but they taste just as good.

CHICKEN RASAM SOUP
SERVES 4

This easy curry is so flavoursome and the peppery sauce goes really well with the pieces of chicken. If you are looking for a delicious soupy vegetarian curry, you could leave the chicken out of this one as the sauce stands perfectly well on its own. It is often served as a vegetarian soup but I like it drizzled over a bowl of steaming hot basmati rice.

PREP TIME: 10 MINS, PLUS
SOAKING TIME
COOKING TIME: 15 MINS

1 golf ball-sized piece of
   tamarind
375ml (1½ cups) hand-hot water
1 level tbsp black peppercorns
1 tsp cumin seeds
2 tsp toor dhal
2 tsp coriander seeds
2 garlic cloves, roughly chopped
1 tsp rapeseed (canola) oil or
   coconut oil
¼ tsp black mustard seeds
3 dried Kashmiri chillies
10 fresh or frozen curry leaves
¼ tsp ground turmeric
200g (7oz) chopped tomatoes
400ml (scant 1¾ cups) cold
   water
400g (14oz) chicken thighs –
   skinned, boned and cut into
   bite-sized pieces
3 tbsp finely chopped coriander
   (cilantro)
Salt, to taste

Add the ball of tamarind to the hot water. Break it up with your hand and allow to soak for about 10 minutes.

Meanwhile, grind the black peppercorns, cumin seeds, toor dhal and coriander seeds to a fine powder using a pestle and mortar or spice grinder. The powder needs to be really fine. Add the garlic and pound it well too.

Heat the oil in a large saucepan over a medium–high heat. When hot, add the mustard seeds. When they begin to pop (after about 30 seconds), reduce the heat to medium and stir in the Kashmiri chillies, curry leaves and ground turmeric. Fry for a further 30 seconds, then tip in the tomatoes and strain in the tamarind water, being careful to ensure that no tamarind seeds make it into the pan. Add the cold water and bring to a boil, then add the chicken and simmer the soup for a further 5–7 minutes, or until the chicken is cooked through. Stir in the coriander and season with salt to taste before serving.

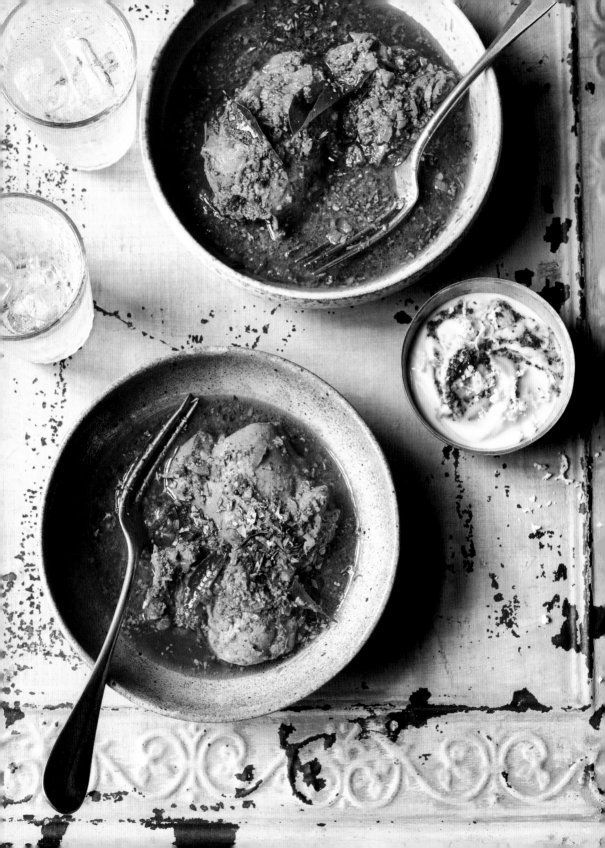

CHICKEN XACUTI

SERVES 4

Chicken xacuti is one of Goa's most famous curries. It is known for its spiciness and its subtle flavour of nutmeg and star anise. It is usually cooked with skinned chicken on the bone, which is what I've done here. If you would like to make it as you get at many British curry houses, use boneless chunks (tikka) of skinned chicken breast or thigh. You can add the meat raw or try pre-cooked tandoori chicken tikka (see page 102). This adds additional layers of flavour and speeds up the final cooking. I wanted to show you this recipe in all its glory. The coconut in this dish increases the fat content, so if you're concerned about fat, reduce the coconut flakes to 35g (½ cup). Me? No way.

PREP TIME: 10 MINS,
PLUS SOAKING TIME
COOKING TIME: 25 MINS

FOR THE XACUTI MASALA

6 dried Kashmiri chillies, chopped (seeds removed for a milder curry)
75g (1 cup) dried coconut flakes
1 tbsp cumin seeds
1 tbsp coriander seeds
1 tsp ajwain (carom) seeds
1 tbsp fennel seeds
1 tbsp black poppy seeds
7 cloves
1 tsp (about 35) black peppercorns
1 cinnamon stick
4 star anise
½ tsp ground turmeric
8 garlic cloves, finely chopped
5cm (2-inch) piece of ginger, peeled and finely chopped

FOR THE CURRY

8 chicken thighs, skinned and on the bone
2 tsp rapeseed (canola) oil
1 tsp black mustard seeds
10 fresh or frozen curry leaves
2 onions, finely chopped
2 green bird's eye chillies, finely chopped
500ml (2 cups) chicken stock or water
1½ tbsp tamarind paste (see page 149) or concentrate
¼ tsp ground nutmeg
20g (¼ cup) coriander (cilantro), chopped
Salt, to taste

Start by making the xacuti masala. In a dry frying pan, toast the Kashmiri chillies for about 1 minute, turning regularly until fragrant. Place in a bowl of warm water to soak for about 30 minutes. Now toast the coconut flakes until lightly browned and set aside. Toast the cumin, coriander, ajwain (carom), fennel and poppy seeds, the cloves, peppercorns, cinnamon stick and star anise over a medium–high heat until fragrant and warm to the touch. Transfer to a bowl and allow to cool.

When the chillies are soft, drain them, reserving the soaking water, then blend them with the coconut flakes and the remaining masala ingredients, along with a little of the chilli soaking water to make a paste, but taste the water first: if it is bitter, use fresh water instead.

Pour the paste over the chicken in a large bowl and mix well to coat. You can start cooking the curry now, but if you would like to marinate the chicken for a couple hours or overnight, it will be even better.

When ready to cook, heat the oil in a large frying pan or wok over a high heat. When bubbles begin to form at the bottom of the pan, add the mustard seeds. When they begin to pop (after about 30 seconds), reduce the heat to medium–high and stir in the curry leaves and let them flavour the oil for about 30 seconds. You'll know when the oil is perfectly flavoured because it will smell so nice. Add the onions and fry for about 5 minutes until soft, lightly browned and translucent. Stir in the chillies and then the chicken and all of the marinade. Stir well to coat the chicken in the onion mixture. Add the stock or water and simmer for about 15 minutes until the chicken is tender and cooked through.

Stir in the tamarind paste or concentrate and nutmeg, then give it a taste. For a sourer flavour, add more tamarind. Nutmeg can taste quite strong to some, but add more if you like. To serve, stir in the coriander and season with salt.

ANDHRA CHICKEN CURRY
SERVES 4

This curry is perfect for those who don't like terribly spicy curries. There are a lot of warming spices in it that produce a delicious flavour, but nothing too fiery-hot. I like the subtle flavour of the fresh mint. If you are pressed for time, you could marinate the meat for just a few minutes and it will still be amazing.

PREP TIME: 10 MINS,
PLUS MARINATING TIME
COOKING TIME: 20 MINS

600g (1lb 5oz) chicken breast,
  cut into bite-sized pieces

FOR THE MARINADE
1 tbsp garlic and ginger paste
¼ tsp ground turmeric
½ tsp salt
2 tbsp lemon juice
2 tbsp low-fat Greek yoghurt
¾ tbsp Kashmiri chilli powder

FOR THE SAUCE
10 cashew nuts, soaked in water
  for 30 minutes
2 tbsp fresh or frozen grated
  coconut (optional)
2 tbsp rapeseed (canola) oil
2–3 cloves
2 cardamom pods, smashed
½ cinnamon stick
½ tsp cumin seeds
10 fresh or frozen curry leaves
3 medium onions, finely
  chopped
1 green chilli, finely chopped
2 tsp garlic and ginger paste
1 tomato, finely chopped
1 tsp Kashmiri chilli powder
  (more or less, to taste)
1 tbsp garam masala (see page
  146)
A handful of mint leaves, finely
  chopped
Salt, to taste

Place all the marinade ingredients in a large mixing bowl and whisk to combine. Rub the marinade into the chicken pieces and leave to stand for at least 20 minutes or overnight for best results. While the chicken is marinating, start working on the sauce. Blend the cashew nuts and coconut (if using) with a drop of water until you have a smooth paste. Set aside.

Heat the oil in a large frying pan or wok over a medium–high heat until visibly hot. Add the cloves, cardamom pods, cinnamon stick, cumin seeds and curry leaves. Allow these ingredients to infuse into the oil for about 30 seconds, then add the onions and green chilli. Fry for about 5 minutes until the onions are soft, translucent and lightly browned. Add the garlic and ginger paste and sizzle for about 30 seconds to cook out the rawness, then stir in the tomato and fry over a medium heat for about 3 minutes until the tomato begins to break down in the sauce. Stir in the chilli powder and garam masala.

Now add the marinated chicken and all the marinade to the pan. Move it around in the onion mixture to coat, then add just enough water to cover (about 350ml/1½ cups). Simmer for about 10 minutes until the chicken is cooked through.

To finish, stir in the mint leaves and cashew paste. Reduce the sauce until you are happy with the consistency and season with salt.

NOTE

If you don't like biting into whole spices like cloves and cardamoms, be sure to count them in and then count them back out before serving. I usually leave them in.

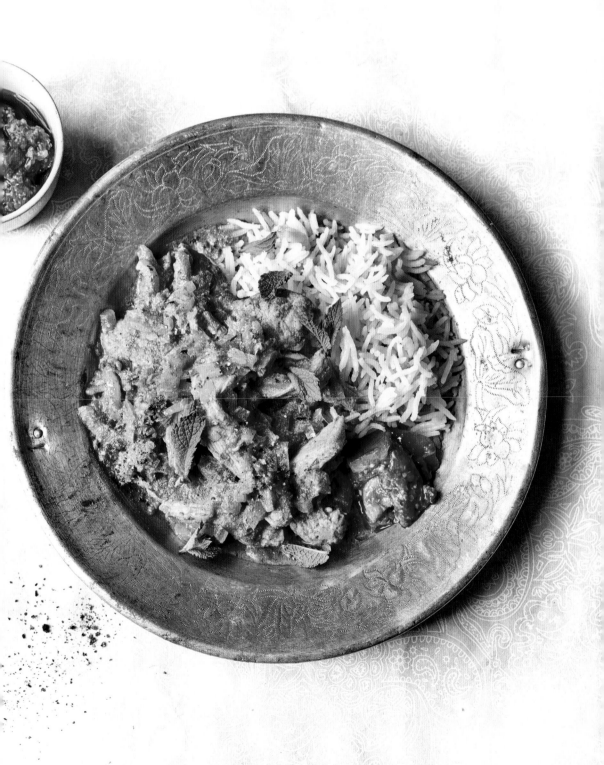

SRI LANKAN BLACK PEPPER CHICKEN CURRY
SERVES 6

One of my favourite curries to this day is the black pepper chicken curry I enjoyed at the restaurant Nuga Gama at The Cinnamon Grand Hotel in Columbo, Sri Lanka. What a place! This is my interpretation of that curry. I believe their version was made with the back bones of chicken and wings that were cut into small pieces. I loved picking up these small bones and gnawing at the meat. It took some work to eat, but it was worth it. All the curries at Nuga Gama were cooked and presented in clay pots. I was determined to do that same. It's not easy carrying a big clay pot back in your hand luggage, but as you can see, I got it back!

PREP TIME: 15 MINS
COOKING TIME: 30 MINS

2 tbsp rapeseed (canola) oil
1 tsp black mustard seeds
1 cinnamon stick
1 tsp cumin seeds
3 cloves
2 bay leaves
About 20 fresh or frozen curry
    leaves
2 onions, finely chopped
3 green chillies (whichever type
    you prefer)
1–2 tbsp finely ground black
    pepper (to taste)
5 green cardamom pods,
    smashed
1 tsp ground turmeric
1 tsp ground cumin
1 tsp ground coriander
1 tsp Kashmiri chilli powder
2 tbsp garlic and ginger paste
1 tbsp soy sauce (this usually
    contains gluten) or tamari
    gluten-free soy sauce
1kg (2lb 4oz) chicken thighs, cut
    into bite-sized pieces
2 sweet green (bell) peppers,
    sliced
20 cherry tomatoes, quartered
1 onion, thinly sliced
400ml (scant 1¾ cups) low-fat
    coconut milk
Salt, to taste

Heat the oil in a large wok or frying pan over a medium–high heat until bubbling hot. Add the mustard seeds and when they begin to crackle (after about 30 seconds), reduce the heat to medium and stir in the cinnamon, cumin seeds, cloves, bay leaves and curry leaves. Add the chopped onions and fry for 6–7 minutes until they begin to turn a light brown colour, then add the green chillies, black pepper and the other ground spices.

Spoon in the garlic and ginger paste and soy sauce and stir to combine. Add the chicken pieces and brown them for about 5 minutes. Add the green peppers, tomatoes and sliced onion and cover the pan. Cook for 5–10 minutes: the chicken and vegetables will release their moisture (a pinch of salt will help with the process).

Pour in the coconut milk and simmer until you are happy with the consistency: this dish can be served either with a lot of sauce or it can be reduced down. Season with salt and perhaps a little more black pepper.

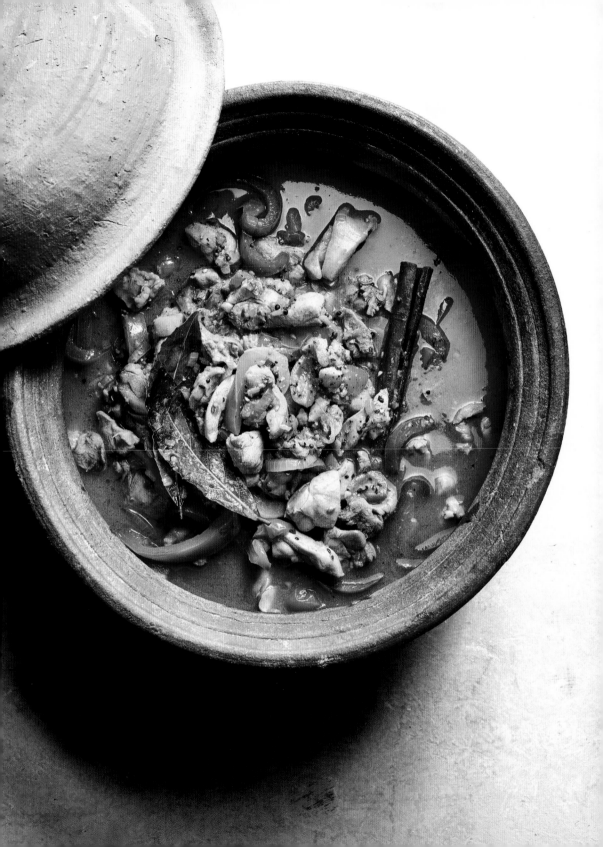

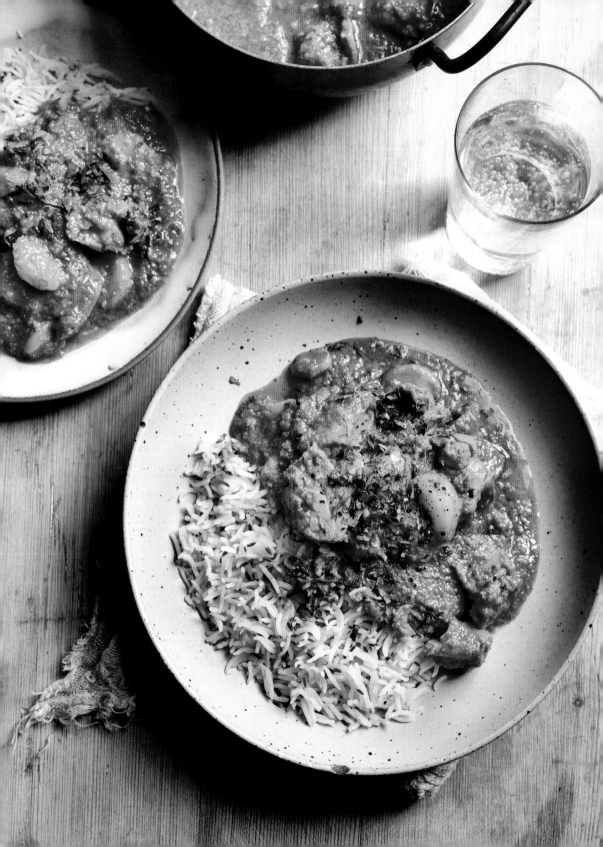

GARLIC & PAPRIKA CHICKEN CURRY

SERVES 4

This one is all about the garlic and paprika! You use a lot of both, but neither overpowers the dish, so don't let the amount of garlic scare you because it mellows as it cooks. The paprika and tomato give the curry a beautiful deep red colour, which looks spicy hot but it's not. Most mild curries at curry houses are quite creamy and can be a bit heavy – no need for cream here. This is one of the healthy, mild curries I used to cook for my kids a lot when they were young. Now they make it for themselves.

PREP TIME: 15 MINS
COOKING TIME: 30 MINS

2 tbsp low-fat Greek yoghurt
2 tbsp smoked sweet paprika
1 tbsp minced ginger
600g (1lb 5oz) chicken thighs, cut into bite-sized pieces
40 garlic cloves, peeled
2 medium onions, chopped
1½ tbsp rapeseed (canola) oil
1 star anise
1 tsp cumin seeds
1 small piece blade mace
5 tinned (canned) anchovy fillets, finely chopped (optional)
½ tsp ground turmeric
250ml (1 cup) tomato purée (see page 146
250ml (1 cup) unsalted chicken stock or water
5 tbsp white wine vinegar or coconut vinegar
Salt, to taste
3 tbsp finely chopped coriander (cilantro)

In a large mixing bowl, whisk the yoghurt with 1 tablespoon of the paprika and the ginger. Stir in the chicken pieces and make sure they are evenly coated in the marinade.

Place half the garlic in a food processor or blender with the onions and about 125ml (½ cup) of water and blend to a thick paste. Set aside.

Heat the oil in a large saucepan or wok over a medium–high heat until visibly hot. Add the whole spices and let them infuse into the oil for about 30 seconds. Add the remaining garlic and the anchovies (if using) and break up the anchovies with a spatula. Fry until the garlic is light brown but not at all burnt. Stir in the onion and garlic paste and the remaining paprika and the turmeric. Now stir in the marinated chicken and the tomato purée. Pour in the stock to cover.

Simmer for 5–10 minutes, or until the chicken is cooked through. Stir in the vinegar and simmer for a further 3 minutes. Season with salt and garnish with the coriander.

NOTE

I often purchase ready-peeled garlic cloves, which is a real timesaver with this dish.

CHETTINAD CHICKEN CURRY
SERVES 4

Don't be scared off by the work needed to make this hugely popular curry. Once the work is done, you will know why I included this recipe in the book. The Chettinad spice masala can be prepared weeks in advance, though it is slightly more intense in flavour if prepared on the day. I often make a large batch of the spice masala to have on hand. With the spice masala at the ready, you can whip this one up fast!

PREP TIME: 15 MINS, PLUS
MARINATING TIME
COOKING TIME: 15 MINS

500g (1lb 2oz) skinned chicken
  breast and/or thighs, cubed

FOR THE MARINADE
½ tsp ground turmeric
¼ tsp Kashmiri chilli powder
Juice of 1 lemon
2 tbsp low-fat Greek yoghurt
2 tbsp garlic and ginger paste

FOR THE CHETTINAD
MASALA
25g (¾oz) fresh or frozen grated
  coconut
8 cashew nuts, soaked in water
  for 30 minutes and tapped dry
2 tsp coriander seeds
2 tsp cumin seeds
1 tsp fennel seeds
10 black peppercorns
Seeds from 3 green cardamom
  pods
3 cloves
½ cinnamon stick, broken into
  small pieces

FOR THE SAUCE
200g (7oz) tinned (canned)
  chopped tomatoes
2 tbsp rapeseed (canola) oil
2 medium onions, very finely
  chopped
¼ tsp ground turmeric
1 tsp Kashmiri chilli powder
15 fresh or frozen curry leaves
Salt, to taste
2 tbsp chopped coriander
  (cilantro)

Whisk all the marinade ingredients in a large bowl and add the chicken. Coat it well and allow to marinate for at least 30 minutes or overnight – the longer the better.

To make the chettinad masala, toast the coconut in a dry frying pan over a medium heat until lightly browned. Transfer to a plate to cool. Do the same with the cashew nuts and transfer to the plate with the coconut. Now toast the remaining masala ingredients until fragrant and warm to the touch but not yet smoking. Transfer to a separate plate to cool, then in a spice grinder or pestle and mortar, grind the toasted whole spices to a fine powder. Add the coconut and cashews and 70ml (¼ cup) of water to make a thick but smooth paste. Set aside.

Now make the sauce. Blend the tomatoes until smooth. Heat the oil in a large frying pan over a medium–high heat and fry the onions for 6–7 minutes until lightly browned. Add the marinated chicken and fry for about 5 minutes, stirring regularly to coat with the fried onions, until almost cooked through. Add the blended tomatoes, the ground turmeric and chilli powder and stir well to combine before adding the chettinad paste and the curry leaves. Allow to sizzle, stirring regularly for another 3 minutes, then pour in 320ml (1¼ cups) of water. Simmer for about 5 minutes until the gravy thickens to your liking (simmer longer for a thicker gravy or if too thick, add a drop more water). Season with salt and garnish with the coriander.

NOTE

This sauce is also good served as a vegetarian/vegan curry. I like it with steamed broccoli and/or cauliflower, but you can add any veggies that sound good to you.

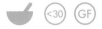

CHICKEN & VEGETABLE STIR-FRY

SERVES 4

This is a straightforward and easy recipe. I love the colour and the different textures. It's a delicious and healthy dish, perfect for cooking up after work.

PREP TIME: 15 MINS, PLUS
MARINATING TIME
COOKING TIME: 15 MINS

500g (1lb 2oz) chicken breast or
  thighs cut into 7mm
  (1¼-inch) slices

FOR THE MARINADE
1½ tbsp lemon juice
¼ tsp ground turmeric
1 tbsp red chilli powder
2 large onions, coarsely pulsed
  in a food mixer
1 tbsp garlic and ginger paste
1 tbsp solid ghee

FOR THE SAUCE
1–2 tbsp rapeseed (canola) oil
1–2 sprigs of curry leaves
2–3 green chillies
1 red onion, thinly sliced
1 red (bell) pepper, seeded and
  thinly sliced
12 cashew nuts, ground into a
  powder
½ tsp freshly ground black
  pepper (or to taste)
12 cherry tomatoes, quartered
2 tbsp garam masala (see page
  146)
Salt, to taste
Coriander (cilantro), to garnish

Mix all the marinade ingredients together in a large bowl, add the chicken and set aside for 20 minutes. Place a wok over a low heat and tip in the chicken with all the marinade. Fry for about 5 minutes until the chicken is cooked through. You can add a couple of tablespoons of water if it looks like the chicken is getting too dry. Once cooked, transfer the chicken and its juices to a bowl and refrigerate until ready to finish the dish.

To make the sauce, heat the oil in a frying pan over a medium heat and add the curry leaves and chillies and fry for about 30 seconds until fragrant. Add the onion and red pepper and fry for about 2 minutes until about half cooked through. Now add the cooked chicken and cook until all the juice is absorbed into the chicken. Add the cashews and black pepper. Continue cooking and stirring to coat the vegetables and chicken with the ground cashew nuts for about 2 minutes until you can smell the cashews. Stir in the tomatoes and season with the garam masala and salt. This is a dry curry, so most of the gravy will be absorbed to give the chicken a succulent texture. Garnish with coriander to serve.

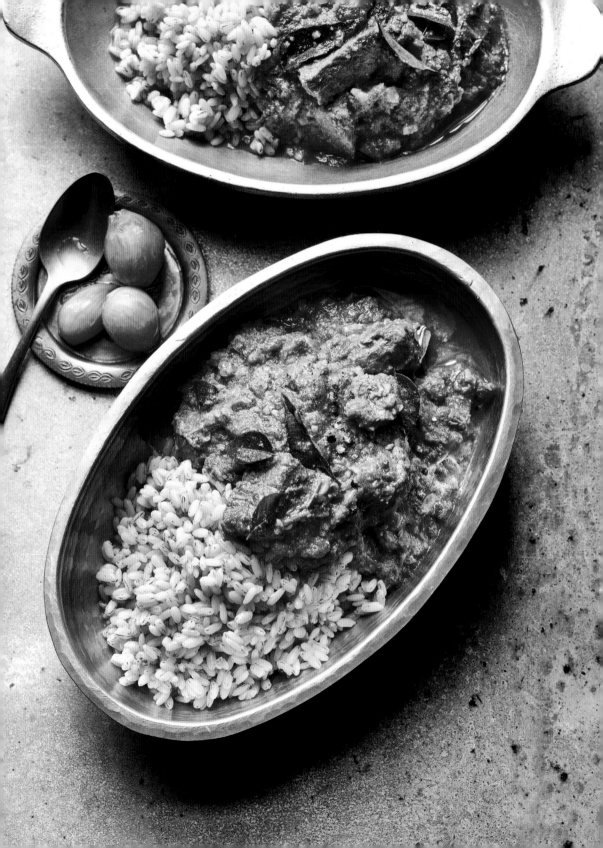

MUTTON MAPPAS
SERVES 6

The first meal I ever ordered in Kerala was mutton mappas. This is so delicious, but a bit difficult to eat as the mutton is cut into small pieces and cooked on the bone until melt-in-the-mouth tender. I love the flavour that the bone-in mutton produces. You need to really get in there with your hands and savour every last bite. Although it looks like a lot of meat, there really isn't much, as most of the weight is in the bones. This curry is a lot like a good stew and the sauce is spectacular spooned over rice, but it can also be eaten just as it comes. Mappas curries are all about the ground coriander, and there's a lot of it in this recipe. You could also make this recipe with lamb or chicken.

PREP TIME: 10 MINS
COOKING TIME: 2½ HOURS

3 tbsp rapeseed (canola) oil
30 fresh or frozen curry leaves
2 red onions, finely chopped
2 green chillies, finely chopped
5cm (2-inch) piece of ginger, peeled and finely chopped
10 garlic cloves, finely chopped
2 tomatoes, diced
1–2 tbsp Kashmiri chilli powder
5 tbsp ground coriander
1 tsp ground turmeric
1 tsp black pepper
1kg (2lb) stewing mutton or lamb cuts on the bone
600ml (2½ cups) light coconut milk
Salt, to taste

Heat the oil in a large saucepan over a medium–high heat until visibly hot. Add about 20 of the curry leaves and infuse them into the oil for about 30 seconds. Add the onions and fry over a medium heat for about 8 minutes, or until light brown in colour. Stir in the green chillies, ginger and garlic, then add the tomatoes and the ground spices.

Add the meat and enough water to cover the meat (about 750ml/ 3 cups) and simmer for 1½ hours or a little longer – the meat is ready when it's ready, so don't rush this! You could add a little more water if needed to cook the meat until tender. It needs to be super-tender, which takes longer with mutton than it does with lamb.

Stir in the coconut milk and season with salt.

NOTE

Many Asian butchers will have exactly the meat cuts you need, as it is required often by their customers. Just ask for small chunks of mutton or lamb on the bone for curries. Of course, if you don't like the idea of picking up the saucy meat on the bone with your hands, you could just use cubed lamb or mutton off the bone.

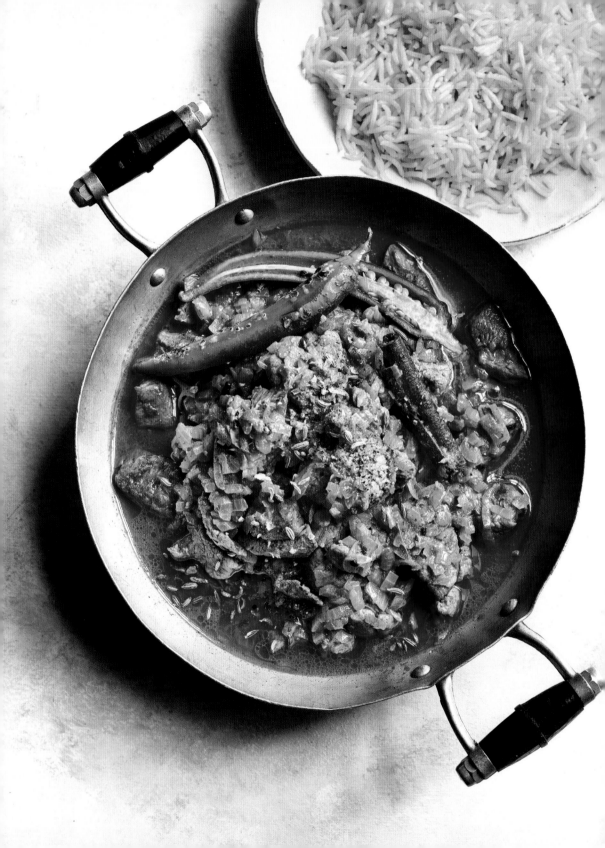

KATTA LAMB CURRY
SERVES 4

Katta lamb curry is truly unique in flavour and mouth-wateringly gorgeous too. What makes it different is the tangy amchoor (dried mango powder) and crushed fennel seeds that are stirred into the sauce at the end of cooking. I usually add a whole lamb leg, cubed, when making this curry and then fish out some of the cooked meat, which I freeze to have on hand for quick lamb BIR (British Indian Restaurant)-style curries. I like to serve this with rice, cauliflower rice or masala chapattis.

PREP TIME: 15 MINS
COOKING TIME: 80 MINS

2 tbsp mustard oil
½ cinnamon stick
1½ tsp cumin seeds
3 cloves
5 green cardamom pods, smashed
3 onions, finely chopped
2 tbsp garlic and ginger paste
1 tsp ground turmeric
1 tsp garam masala (see page 146)
½ tsp Kashmiri chilli powder
500g (1lb 2oz) lean lamb, cut into bite-sized pieces
3 heaped tsp amchoor (dried mango powder)
1½ tsp fennel seeds, lightly crushed
2 tsp dried fenugreek leaves (kasoori methi)
3 green chillies, cut lengthways
Salt, to taste
Chopped coriander (cilantro), to garnish

Heat the oil in a saucepan or wok over a medium–high heat until visibly hot. Add the cinnamon, cumin seeds, cloves and cardamom pods. Remember that if you don't like biting into whole spices, count them in and then count them back out again before serving. Temper the spices in the oil for about 30 seconds, then add the onions and fry for about 5 minutes until soft, translucent and lightly browned.

Stir in the garlic and ginger paste and fry for a further minute, then add the turmeric, garam masala, chilli powder and lamb. Stir well to combine. Add about 300ml (1¼ cups) of water, cover the pan and simmer on a medium heat for about 1 hour, or until the meat is really tender.

Stir in the amchoor (dried mango powder), fennel seeds, dried fenugreek (kasoori methi) and green chillies. Continue to simmer until you are happy with the consistency of the sauce. Season with salt and garnish with the coriander.

PORK BAFAT
SERVES 4

This recipe is popular with the Christian population in Goa. It can also be made with chicken. I really like the spicy flavour of the bafat curry powder (see page 149) together with the sharp taste of the vinegar. This is gorgeous over matta rice (see page 123) but it is also nice served on its own, as the sweet potato can be quite filling.

PREP TIME: 15 MINS
(INCLUDES MAKING THE
BAFAT CURRY POWDER)
COOKING TIME: 30 MINS

1 golf ball-sized piece of tamarind or 1 tsp tamarind paste (see page 149) or concentrate
2 tbsp bafat curry powder (see page 149)
2 tbsp rapeseed (canola) oil
1 cinnamon stick
6 cloves
2 onions, finely chopped
3 tbsp garlic and ginger paste
3 green bird's eye chillies, cut into thin rings
800g (1lb 12oz) lean pork cut into 1cm (½-inch) cubes
4 tbsp malt vinegar (more or less, to taste)
1 sweet potato, cut into cubes the same size as the pork (optional)
Salt, to taste

Heat 250ml (1 cup) of water until coffee-hot. Add the tamarind, give it a good stir and set aside. For best results use block tamarind.

Place the bafat curry powder in a mixing bowl with 125ml (½ cup) of water. Stir well to combine, then set aside.

Heat the oil a large saucepan over a medium–high heat until visibly hot. Add the cinnamon stick and cloves and let the spices infuse into the oil for about 30 seconds. Add the onions and fry over a medium heat for about 5 minutes, or until soft and translucent. Stir in the garlic and ginger paste and the chillies and fry for a further 30 seconds.

Stir the curry/water mixture into the onions. Fry over a medium heat for a further 5 minutes. If it is looking too dry, add a drop more water so that the spices don't burn. Add the pork, 250ml (1 cup) of water and the vinegar. Stir well, then cover the pan. This curry doesn't have a lot of sauce and more liquid will be cooked out of the pork to make a delicious, thick gravy. Cook on a medium heat for about 10 minutes, stirring from time to time. Add the sweet potato (if using) and the tamarind water. If using block tamarind, strain the water through a sieve or use your hand so that all you pour into the pan is tamarind water with no solids. Cover again and cook for a further 10 minutes, or until the sweet potato is cooked through. Check for seasoning and add salt before serving if needed.

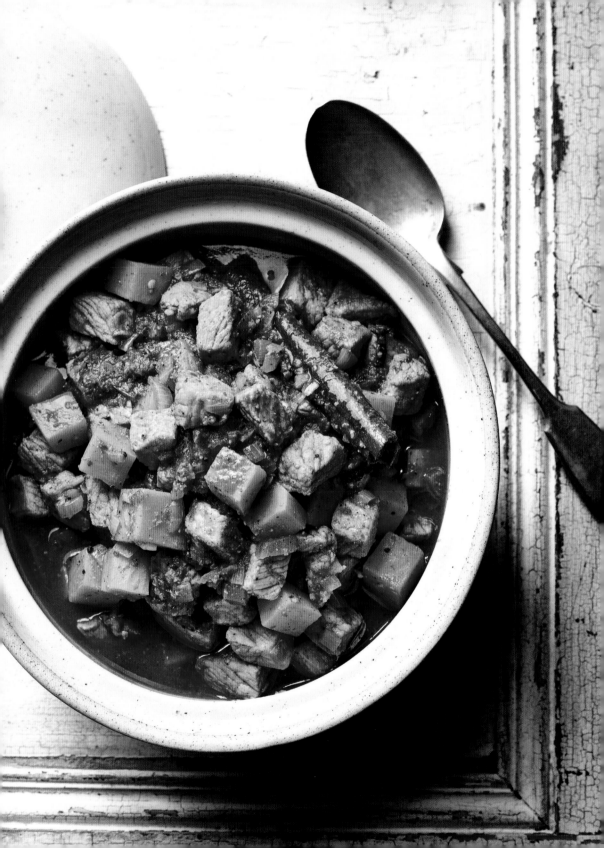

GOAN BEEF KOFTA CURRY
SERVES 4

I have to say I do love kofta curries. These beef koftas are simmered in light coconut milk, which flavours the sauce. If you can't purchase beef mince that has been ground twice, you could knead it for a couple of minutes to break it down. It is also nice with lean chicken mince. The sauce is really flavourful, so the curry can also be made with vegetarian koftas, using a recipe like the corn and potato seekh kebabs on page 111. If using vegetarian koftas, add them right at the end of cooking.

PREP TIME: 10 MINS
COOKING TIME: 20 MINS

500g (1lb 12oz) lean beef mince (ask your butcher to grind it twice)
1 tbsp ground cumin
1 tsp ground coriander
2 tsp chilli powder
1 tsp flaky salt
1 tbsp freshly ground black pepper
4 tbsp garlic and ginger paste
1 egg
1 tbsp coconut oil or rapeseed (canola) oil
1 tsp black mustard seeds
10 fresh or frozen curry leaves
2 medium onions, finely chopped
3 tbsp finely sliced garlic
2 green chillies, finely chopped
½ tsp ground turmeric
400g (14oz) tinned (canned) chopped tomatoes
400ml (scant 1¾ cups) light coconut milk
2 tbsp soy sauce (this usually contains gluten), tamari gluten-free soy sauce or coconut amino
Salt, to taste
Coriander (cilantro), chopped, to serve

Start by making the koftas. In a large bowl, mix the mince with the cumin, ground coriander, 1 teaspoon of the chilli powder, the salt, black pepper, garlic and ginger paste, and egg. Knead well so that all the ingredients are mixed into the meat. Form into 16 small, golf ball-sized koftas, cover and refrigerate until ready to cook.

Heat the oil in a large frying pan over a high heat until visibly hot. Add the mustard seeds and when they begin to crackle (after about 30 seconds), reduce the temperature to medium–high, stir in the curry leaves and fry until fragrant – about 30 seconds should do nicely.

Add the onions and fry for about 5 minutes until soft and translucent. Stir in the garlic and chillies and fry for a further minute or so. Add the turmeric and stir well. Pour in the tomatoes, coconut milk and soy sauce or coconut amino.

Place the koftas in the sauce and simmer for about 10 minutes until cooked through. Check for seasoning and add more salt if needed. Garnish with coriander and serve.

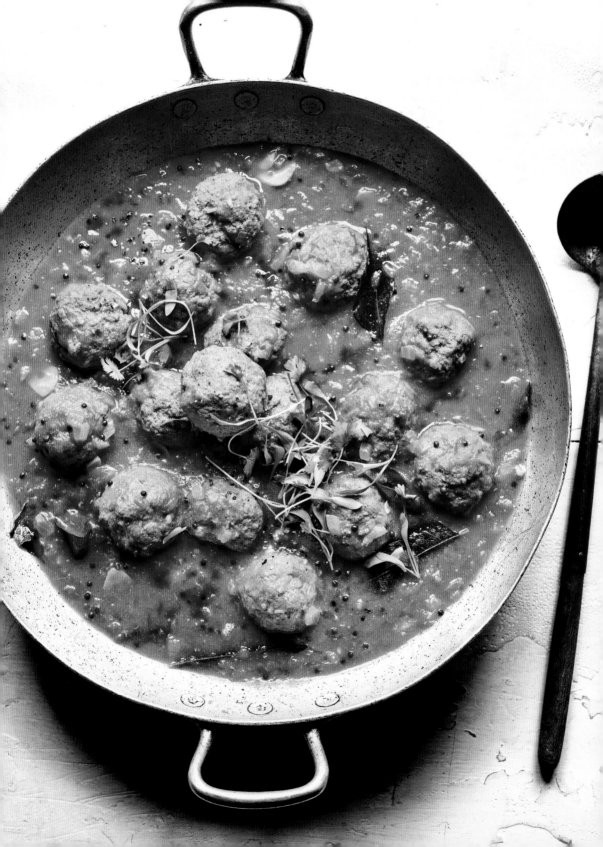

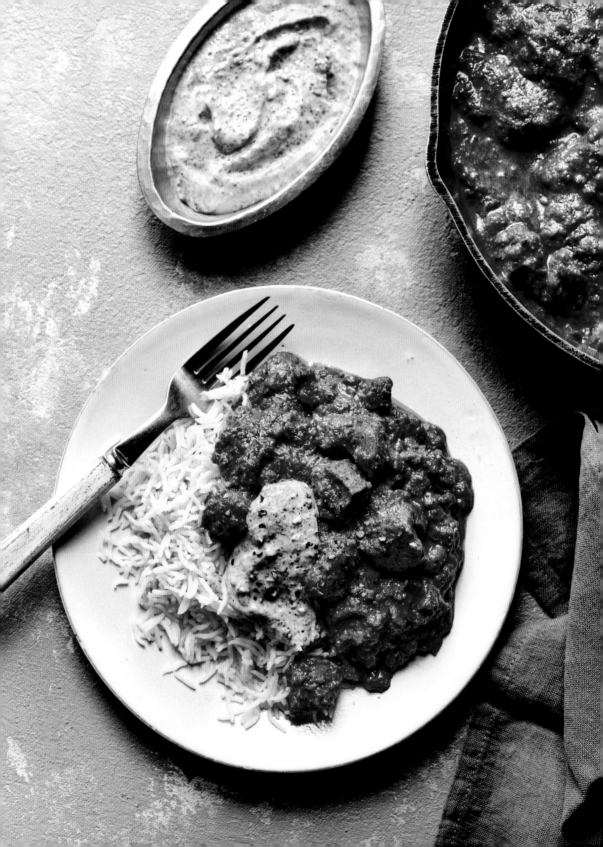

VENISON ROGAN JOSH

SERVES 4

I've been a big fan of venison since I was about ten. My grandfather used to make some amazing venison stews that were slowly cooked for hours until the meat literally fell apart in your mouth. I remember spooning the sauce and meat over polenta and never wanting the meal to end. Rogan josh is usually made with lamb or mutton, but this venison version simply has to be tried. Cook it on a day when you have a lot of time as the meat really does need to cook a good long time. Venison has half the fat of lamb and mutton but spectacular flavour. Just don't rush things... it's ready when it's ready.

PREP TIME: 30 MINS, PLUS
MARINATING TIME
COOKING TIME: 2½ HOURS

150g (5½oz) fat-free Greek
    yoghurt
3 generous tbsp ground almonds
3 tbsp garlic and ginger paste
A pinch of saffron (about 10
    threads)
600g (1lb 5oz) lean venison meat
Seeds from 10 green cardamom
    pods (4½ tbsp)
1 cinnamon stick
1 star anise
2 blades of mace
2 tbsp cumin seeds
3 tbsp coriander seeds
1 tbsp black peppercorns
½ tsp ground turmeric
2 tbsp rapeseed (canola) oil
3 medium onions, finely
    chopped
1 tbsp sweet or hot paprika (you
    decide)
2 tbsp tomato purée (see page
    146)
Salt, to taste
Coriander and chilli raita (see
    page 136), to serve (optional)

Whisk the yoghurt, ground almonds, 1 tablespoon of the garlic and ginger paste, and the saffron together in a large bowl. Cut the venison into small, bite-sized pieces and stir it into the marinade so that the meat is coated all over. Leave to marinate in the fridge for at least 2 hours, though overnight or up to three days is even better.

When ready to cook, toast the whole spices in a dry frying pan until fragrant and warm to the touch but not smoking. Transfer to a plate to cool and grind to a fine powder. Stir in the ground turmeric and set aside.

Heat the oil in a large saucepan or wok and fry the onions for about 5 minutes until translucent and lightly browned. Stir in the meat to brown it. If the onions and meat appear to be sticking to the pan, add 1–2 tablespoons of water, but don't be tempted to add more: you want to sear the meat but not boil it yet. Stir in the remaining garlic and ginger paste.

Add the paprika, ground spice blend, tomato purée and about 500ml (2 cups) of water. Simmer for about 2 hours or longer if necessary. You will know when the curry is ready because the meat will be fall-apart gorgeous!

Season with salt before serving and top with homemade coriander and chilli raita if you like.

TURKEY KEEMA WITH PEAS
SERVES 4

Any minced meat can be used in this recipe. Keema is usually made with lamb, mutton, goat or beef, but here I have used turkey, which is, of course, a low-calorie option. The turkey is quite flavourful with all the spices and other ingredients, but you might prefer to use low-fat beef instead. It will be slightly higher in calories though. Many people have asked me how to make keema like the smooth saucy keema you find at good takeaways and restaurants. Add water to the meat as described below and you will love how it turns out.

PREP TIME: 10 MINS
COOKING TIME: 20 MINS

500g (1lb 2oz) lean turkey mince
500ml (2 cups) water
2 tbsp rapeseed (canola) oil
1 tsp cumin seeds
6 green cardamom pods, smashed
½ cinnamon stick
6 black peppercorns
3 medium onions (about 500g/1lb 2oz), finely chopped
2 tbsp garlic and ginger paste
1–3 green chillies, finely chopped
½ tsp chilli powder
½ tsp ground cumin
½ tsp garam masala (see page 146)
100ml (3½fl oz) tomato purée (see page 146)
150g (5½oz) fresh or frozen peas
Salt, to taste

Begin by preparing the minced meat. Place the mince in a large bowl and pour the water over it. Stir well with a fork until the meat has soaked up all the water – it should be about the same consistency as cooked oatmeal. Set aside.

Heat the oil in a frying pan over a medium–high heat until visibly hot. Add the cumin seeds, cardamom pods, cinnamon stick and black peppercorns and let these spices temper in the oil for about 30 seconds. Add the onions and sauté for 5–7 minutes until soft, translucent and lightly browned. Add the garlic and ginger paste and fry for about 30 seconds, then add the green chillies and fry for a further minute. Now add the mince and fry for about 5 minutes to brown.

Add the ground spices and tomato purée. Stir in the peas and simmer for about 3 minutes until cooked through. Season with salt and serve.

BINDI GOSHT

SERVES 4

As with any meat curry, this one is ready when it's ready. You need to let the lamb cook low and slow! When it is tender and the sauce very tasty, it's ready to serve. You will notice that I have used very little meat here so that you can eat light but still get the fantastic flavour of lamb. When preparing okra, you need to take care that it doesn't become slimy. There are a couple of ways you can avoid this. Firstly, you can soak the whole okra in vinegar for 30 minutes before rinsing and drying it and using in the dish, or secondly, you can freeze the okra before using it. Once you have trimmed the okra, it should be cooked immediately for best results.

PREP TIME: 10 MINS
COOKING TIME: 45–60 MINS

2 tbsp rapeseed (canola) oil
1 cinnamon stick
1 tsp cumin seeds
Seeds from 2 black or 4 green cardamom pods
2 medium onions, grated
400g (14oz) lean stewing lamb, diced
400g (14oz) tinned (canned) chopped tomatoes
½ tsp ground cloves
1 tbsp ground coriander
1 tbsp garam masala (see page 146)
1 tsp chilli powder
20 okra, ends cut off
Salt, to taste

Heat the oil over a medium–high heat in a saucepan until visibly hot. Add the cinnamon stick, cumin seeds and cardamom seeds. Temper these spices in the oil for about 30 seconds, then add the onions and fry for 5 minutes until just beginning to turn a light brown. Stir in the lamb and brown for about 3 minutes.

Add the tomatoes and ground spices and top with about 250ml (1 cup) of water. Simmer for 45 minutes. If the meat is not yet tender after 45 minutes, continue cooking until it is. You might need to add a little more water during cooking. When the meat is tender, stir in the okra and cook for a further 5 minutes, or until the okra is soft. Season with salt and serve.

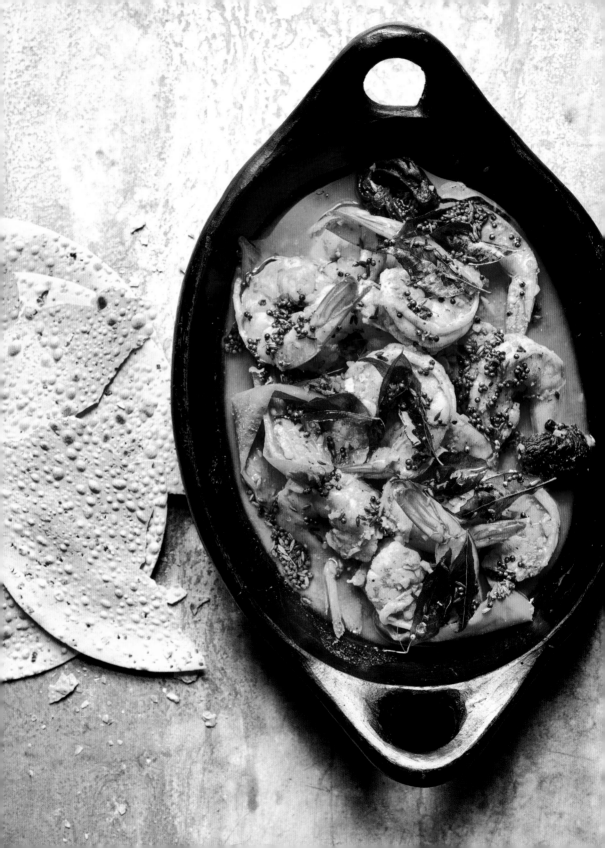

KERALAN PRAWN CURRY
SERVES 4

This has to be one of the easiest curries I've ever made! In Kerala, kokum is often used as a souring agent with seafood curries instead of tamarind, which is also popular. In this recipe I use kokum (see suppliers on page 156) but if you have trouble sourcing it, just add the suggested amount of shop-bought tamarind concentrate or make your own paste (see page 149). I demonstrate this curry at many of my cooking classes and it always goes down well. Many people have said they wouldn't think about making it if they saw it in a cookbook because it seems so strange. Taste the sharp and tart flavour of that kokum sauce and you'll be hooked! It's so good, unique and simply delicious. This dish is fantastic served with matta rice (see page 123) and/or papadams.

PREP TIME: 5 MINS
COOKING TIME: 25 MINS

1 tsp Kashmiri chilli powder
½ tsp ground turmeric
1 tbsp ground coriander
½ tsp freshly ground black pepper
2.5cm (1-inch) piece of ginger, peeled and finely minced
5 green chillies, sliced down the middle
3 kokums or 2 tsp tamarind paste (see page 149) or concentrate
500g (1lb 2oz) medium raw prawns, shelled and cleaned
3 garlic cloves, minced
1–1½ tbsp rapeseed (canola) oil or coconut oil
1 tsp black mustard seeds
1 tsp cumin seeds
20 fresh or frozen curry leaves
Salt, to taste

Pour 500ml (2 cups) of water in a saucepan and bring to the boil. Stir in the Kashmiri chilli powder, turmeric, coriander, black pepper, ginger, green chillies and kokums and simmer for 15 minutes. Add the prawns, cover with a lid and simmer for about 5 minutes. Uncover the pan and stir in the garlic and stir well to combine.

Heat the oil in a small frying pan over a medium–high heat until visibly hot, then add the mustard seeds. When they start to crackle (after about 30 seconds), add the cumin seeds and curry leaves. Allow to infuse into the oil for about 30 seconds, then pour over the cooked prawns. Season with salt and serve hot.

NOTE

The kokum pieces are not meant to be eaten. They are edible but they are very sour.

GOAN PRAWN CURRY
SERVES 4

In my opinion, this one has to be made with small prawns. I've had it with large prawns too, but the baby, bite-sized prawns just do it for me. If you're a calorie counter, no need to worry here – prawns are very low in calories. If you wish, the sauce could be made even lighter by halving the amount of grated coconut with not much loss of flavour. This is great served with white or brown rice or the cauliflower rice pilau on page 124.

PREP TIME: 15 MINS, PLUS
SOAKING TIME
COOKING TIME: 15 MINS

FOR THE PASTE
4 pieces of dried kokum★
½ tsp cumin seeds
2 tbsp coriander seeds
10 Kashmiri chillies (remove the
    seeds for a milder curry)
150g (5½oz) fresh or frozen
    grated coconut
6 garlic cloves

FOR THE CURRY
1–2 tbsp rapeseed (canola) oil
10 fresh or frozen curry leaves
1 red onion, finely sliced and cut
    into 2.5cm (1-inch) pieces
2 green bird's eye chillies, slit
    lengthways
600g (1lb 5oz) small raw prawns
2 medium tomatoes, quartered
Salt, to taste
3 tbsp finely chopped coriander
    (cilantro)

Soak the kokum in 250ml (1 cup) of hot water for about 20 minutes.

To make the paste, heat a dry frying pan over a medium–high heat and toast the cumin seeds and coriander seeds for 2 minutes until fragrant and warm to the touch. Transfer to a bowl to cool. Toast the Kashmiri chillies until warm to the touch, being careful not to blacken them. Allow to cool with the cumin and coriander.

Toast the coconut until fragrant and deep brown in colour. Transfer to the bowl with the spices to cool. Once cooled, blend the kokum pieces with the garlic and toasted ingredients into a paste with about 250ml (1 cup) of water.

In a large high-sided frying pan or saucepan, heat the oil over a medium–high heat until visibly hot. Add the curry leaves and let them temper in the oil for about 30 seconds. Add the onion and fry for 5–7 minutes until soft and translucent and beginning to turn a light brown. Stir in the green chillies, the spice paste and the prawns. Add just enough water to cover (about 250ml/1 cup) and simmer until the prawns are cooked through – don't over-cook them or they will become hard – just a few minutes should be enough.

Just as the prawns are about ready, add the tomatoes and stir it all up to combine. Season with salt and sprinkle with the coriander.

★You could substitute the dried kokum with 2–3 teaspoons of tamarind paste (see page 149) or concentrate, or to taste. If you can't get tamarind, squeeze a little lime juice over the finished dish just before serving.

PRAWN & RAW MANGO CURRY

SERVES 4

This simple curry is one you've got try. It might be easy to make, but this special combination of ingredients tastes like you've been slaving over a hot stove all day! The sweet raw mango gives this curry an exotic flavour that makes me want to cook it all the time. This curry has a rather thin sauce that is delicious spooned over hot white rice. If you're not concerned about fat content, try increasing the coconut to 100g (about half a coconut) for a richer taste. If you can take the heat, use a little more chilli powder than suggested in the recipe.

PREP TIME: 15 MINS
COOKING TIME: 15 MINS

65g (2¼oz) fresh or frozen grated coconut
2½ tbsp rapeseed (canola) oil or coconut oil
1 tsp fennel seeds
3 shallots, finely sliced
1 tsp brown mustard seeds
15 fresh or frozen curry leaves
1 large onion, finely chopped
2–3 green chillies, sliced down the middle
1½ tbsp garlic and ginger paste
1 tsp Kashmiri chilli powder
1½ tbsp ground coriander
½ tsp ground cumin
½ tsp ground turmeric
¼ tsp ground fenugreek
1 mango, stoned and thinly sliced
250g (9oz) shelled raw prawns
Salt, to taste

Heat a dry frying pan over a medium heat and toast the coconut until light brown. Add ½ teaspoon of the oil and the fennel seeds and shallots and stir to combine. Fry for a further minute, then remove from the heat and grind to a fine paste in a spice grinder or pestle and mortar.

Using the same pan, add the remaining oil and heat it over a medium–high heat. When hot, add the mustard seeds. When they begin to pop (after about 30 seconds), add the curry leaves and sizzle for about 30 seconds.

Add the onion, reduce the heat to medium and fry for 5–6 minutes until soft and translucent. Add the green chillies and the garlic and ginger paste and fry for a further minute, then stir in the chilli powder, coriander, cumin, turmeric, fenugreek and mango.

Stir well and add 250ml (1 cup) of water and the prawns and simmer for 5 minutes until the prawns are just cooked through. Add the coconut mixture and stir in a little more water (up to 250ml/1 cup) for a thinner, soupier sauce. When you are happy with the consistency, season with salt and serve.

KERALAN CRAB ROAST

SERVES 4

I've had this dish many times in India where the crabs are small and sweet. This makes for a beautiful presentation, as you can see from the frozen crabs I used in the photograph opposite. The fresh crabs we get off the coast of the UK are much larger, but their flavour is equally delicious. You could source small Indian crabs both online or from specialist shops, but any crab will do! Try this with cracked, locally sourced crab claws and you won't be disappointed. This is a fun recipe to serve to a group – just get stuck in and be prepared to get your hands dirty. A little plain basmati rice, matta rice (see page 123) or cauliflower rice (see page 124) served with this curry is all you need.

PREP TIME: 10 MINS
COOKING TIME: 15 MINS

2 tbsp rapeseed (canola) oil or coconut oil
15 fresh or frozen curry leaves
1½ tsp Kashmiri chilli powder
1 tsp ground coriander
½ tsp ground turmeric
½ tsp dried red pepper flakes
1 onion, finely chopped
2 tbsp garlic and ginger paste
1 green chilli, sliced down the middle
2 pieces of dried kokum (or see substitutes on page 11)
4 cooked small brown crabs (available at most fishmongers) or the equivalent in cracked crab claws or any crab of your choice
125ml (½ cup) water
Salt and freshly ground black pepper, to taste
3 tbsp finely chopped coriander (cilantro), to garnish

Heat the oil in a large wok or high-sided frying pan over a medium–high heat until visibly hot. Add 10 curry leaves and sauté them for about 30 seconds until fragrant. Add the Kashmiri chilli powder, ground coriander, turmeric and dried red pepper flakes and give it all a good stir to combine.

Now add the onion and fry for 5–7 minutes until translucent and light brown in colour. Add the garlic and ginger paste, green chilli, kokum, crabs and the water. Bring to a simmer and cook over a low heat until the crab is heated through and the water has reduced by about half – about 8 minutes should do. Check for seasoning and add salt if needed. Throw in the remaining curry leaves for added flavour just before serving.

Check for seasoning, adding salt and black pepper if needed, and garnish with the coriander.

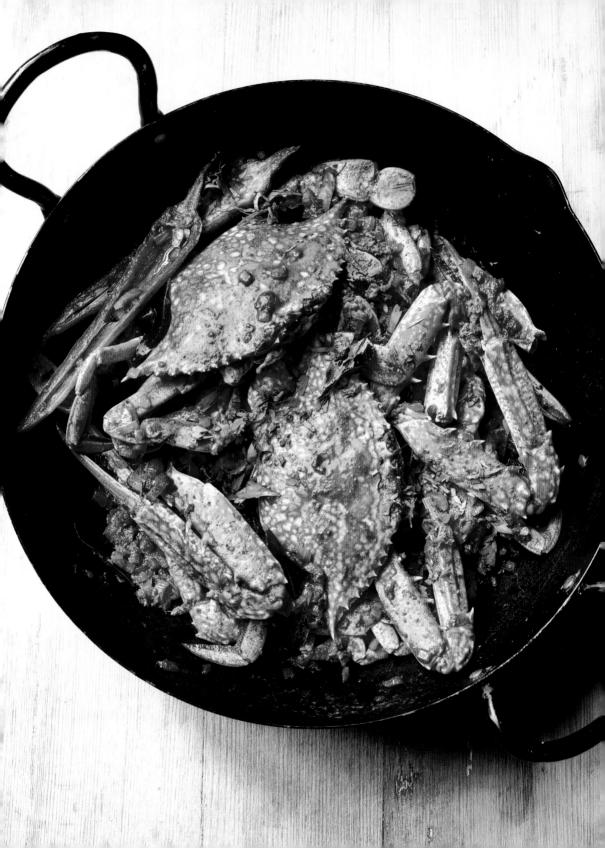

214KCAL

12.2G CARBS

MULAKITTATHU FISH CURRY

SERVES 4

This is one of my favourite seafood curries. The kokum can be substituted with tamarind paste (see page 146) or concentrate, but do try to find it! For me, the flavour of the stewed kokum makes this dish. In Kerala, the curry is usually made with kingfish, which is difficult to find in the UK. I used cod and found it to be equally delicious. Mulakittathu curry is often fiery hot. I toned it down for my family as they prefer their curries milder! Feel free to use more Kashmiri chilli powder and omit the paprika. These two spices are what gives the curry its characteristic red colour.

PREP TIME: 10 MINS
COOKING TIME: 20 MINS

3 kokums or 2 tsp tamarind
   paste (see page 149) or
   concentrate
1½ tbsp rapeseed (canola) oil or
   coconut oil
½ tsp fenugreek seeds
20 fresh or frozen curry leaves,
   plus extra to garnish
2 red onions, finely chopped
7 garlic cloves, thinly sliced
2.5cm (1-inch) piece of ginger,
   peeled and minced
3 green bird's eye chillies, sliced
   lengthways
1 tbsp Kashmiri chilli powder
1 tbsp sweet paprika
1 generous tbsp ground
   coriander
½ tsp ground turmeric
200g (7oz) chopped tomatoes
500g (1lb 2oz) cod, cut into bite-
   sized pieces
Salt, to taste
Coriander (cilantro), to garnish

If using kokums, wash and then soak them in 400ml (scant 1¾ cups) of water until needed.

Heat the oil in a large saucepan over a medium–high heat until visibly hot. Add the fenugreek seeds and curry leaves and let these infuse into the oil for about 30 seconds. Add the onions and fry for about 5 minutes until lightly browned. Stir in the garlic, ginger and chillies and fry for a further minute, then add the Kashmiri chilli powder, paprika, ground coriander and ground turmeric and stir to combine.

Add the tomatoes, the kokums with the water they were soaked in or 2 tsp tamarind paste or concentrate, and 400ml (scant 1¾ cups) of water. Bring to the boil and simmer for 5 minutes. Then add the fish and cook, covered, over a medium heat for 10–15 minutes, or until the fish is just cooked through. A little more water could be added if you prefer a thinner sauce. Stir in a handful more curry leaves (optional), then season with salt and garnish with coriander before serving.

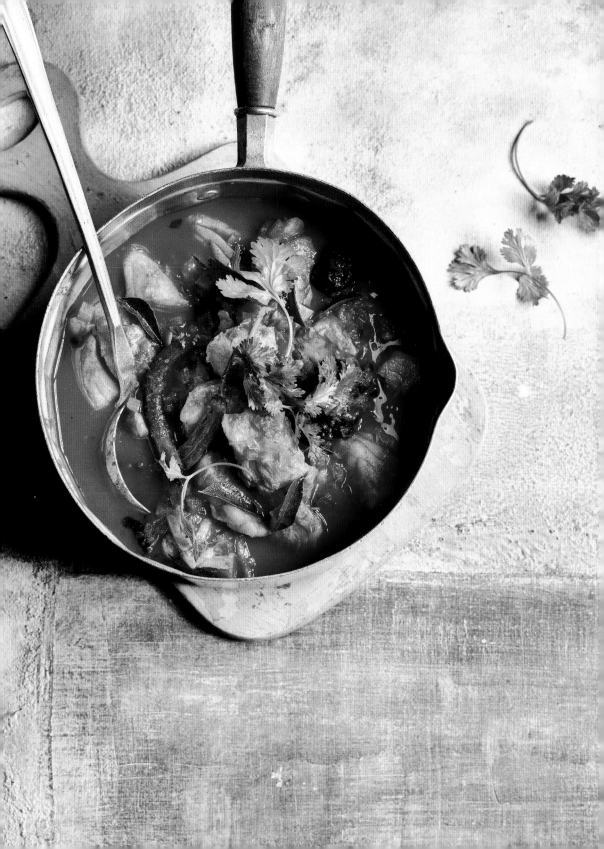

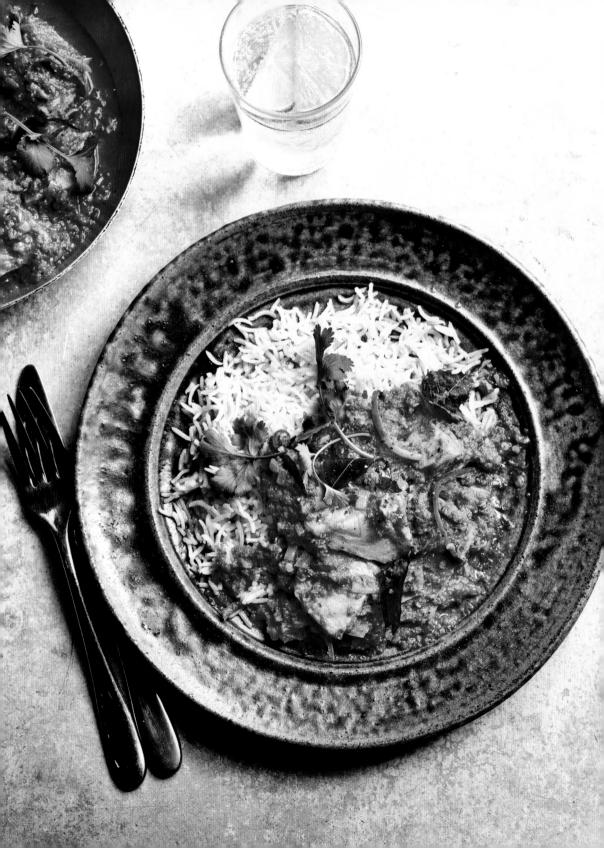

SWORDFISH AMBOT TIK

SERVES 4

The way I have had this curry most often is with baby shark, which I really love. It's caught right off the coast of Goa. It did make me think when I jumped into the sea – they aren't man eaters, but they could certainly take off a toe if they wanted. Shark isn't very easy to find in the UK, so I have substituted another of my favourite fish, swordfish. This dish is great served simply with the rice of your choice.

PREP TIME: 15 MINS
COOKING TIME: 10 MINS

1 tsp flaky sea salt
500g (1lb 2oz) swordfish,
   skinned and thickly sliced
2 tbsp coconut oil or rapeseed
   (canola) oil
10 fresh or frozen curry leaves
1 medium onion, finely chopped
200g (7oz) chopped tomatoes
2 green chillies, sliced
   lengthways
1–2 tbsp tamarind paste (see
   page 149) or concentrate
Salt, to taste
Coriander (cilantro), to garnish

FOR THE PASTE

10 dried Kashmiri chillies
1 medium red onion, roughly
   chopped
6 large garlic cloves, smashed
2.5cm (1-inch) piece of ginger,
   peeled and roughly chopped
1 tsp cumin seeds
6 cloves, smashed
$\frac{1}{2}$ tsp freshly ground black
   pepper
$\frac{1}{4}$ tsp ground turmeric
$\frac{1}{2}$ cinnamon stick

In a bowl, stir the salt into the fish and set aside while you make the sauce.

Blend all the curry paste ingredients together with roughly 70ml ($\frac{1}{4}$ cup) of water to make a thick, smooth paste. Set aside.

Heat the oil in a large saucepan or wok over a medium–high heat until visibly hot. Add the curry leaves and temper them in the oil for about 30 seconds, then add the onion and fry for 5–7 minutes until lightly browned.

Add the curry paste and tomatoes and give it all a good stir. Now add enough water to make a gravy that is to your preferred consistency – I used about 250ml (1 cup). Add the chillies and the fish and push the fish down into the simmering sauce to cook. It should only take about 3 minutes.

To finish, stir in the tamarind paste or concentrate 1 tablespoon at a time – tamarind gives the curry a nice sour flavour. I recommend tasting the sauce after 1 tablespoon and then adding more if you like. Season with salt and garnish with the coriander.

KARIMEEN POLLICHATHU

SERVES 4

'Karimeen' refers to a type of freshwater fish called pearl spot in English, and 'pollichathu' refers to the fact that it is cooked in a banana leaf. Pearl spot is delicious, but it's difficult to find in the UK, so I usually use salmon or sea trout fillets. I love pearl spot, but I don't think you will be disappointed with this salmon version. Browse the ingredients and it looks like an awful lot of oil being used – only a small amount is actually consumed though. The finished dish is quite red in colour because of the amount of chilli powder used. Use less if you don't like your food spicy, or add sweet paprika. I learned this recipe from my friend Rahul Krishnan Muttumpuram, Executive Chef at Cheenavala Seafood Restaurant in Kochi.

PREP TIME: 10 MINS,
PLUS MARINATING TIME
COOKING TIME: 10 MINS

1 tbsp lime juice
1 tsp ground turmeric
1 tbsp Kashmiri chilli powder
1 tsp black pepper
½ tsp fennel powder or a few
    seeds crushed into a powder
½ tsp flaky sea salt
600g (1lb 5oz) salmon or sea
    trout fillet
100ml (3½fl oz) coconut oil or
    rapeseed (canola) oil
1 tsp garlic and ginger paste
6 medium shallots, thinly sliced
10 fresh or frozen curry leaves
½ tomato, diced
1 tsp tamarind paste (see page
    149) or concentrate
1 tbsp thick coconut milk
1 small red onion, cut into thin
    rings, to garnish
Lime wedges, to garnish

You will need a banana leaf, or
    foil, if you can't get hold of
    one.

In a large bowl, whisk the lime juice, ground turmeric, Kashmiri chilli powder, black pepper, fennel powder and salt together, then add the fish fillet. Be sure to completely cover the fish with the marinade and set aside for 20 minutes.

Heat about 1 teaspoon of the oil in a frying pan over a medium–high heat. Remove the salmon from the marinade and sear on both sides for about 2 minutes, then set aside.

To make the masala sauce, heat 1½ tablespoons of the oil in a separate frying pan over a medium–high heat and add the garlic and ginger paste, shallots, curry leaves and tomato and sauté for 2 minutes until the shallots turn soft. Pour in the excess marinade from the fish and sauté for a further 2–4 minutes, being careful not to burn the garlic or spices. Stir in the tamarind paste or concentrate and coconut milk, then add the seared salmon fillet. Move the fish around in the masala so that is nicely coated.

Now take a banana leaf (foil can be substituted if necessary) and tie the fish and all the masala into a packet using a piece of string. Clean the pan and heat the remaining oil over a medium heat. Place the wrapped salmon in the oil and cook the fish packet on both sides for about 2–3 minutes, or a little longer if you don't like your salmon pink in the middle.

To serve, open the packet and garnish with the sliced onion rings and lime wedges.

NOTE

The salmon packet is also nice cooked on a grill over hot coals on the barbecue.

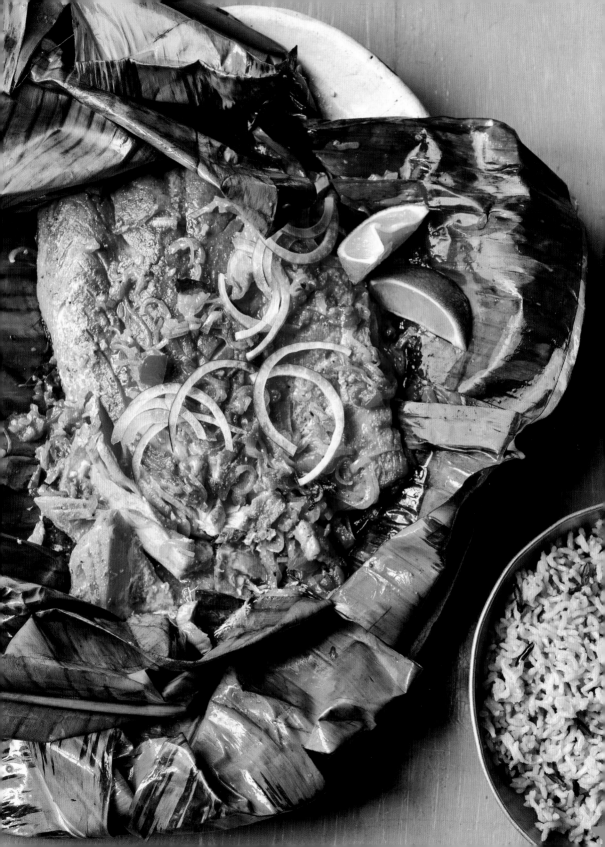

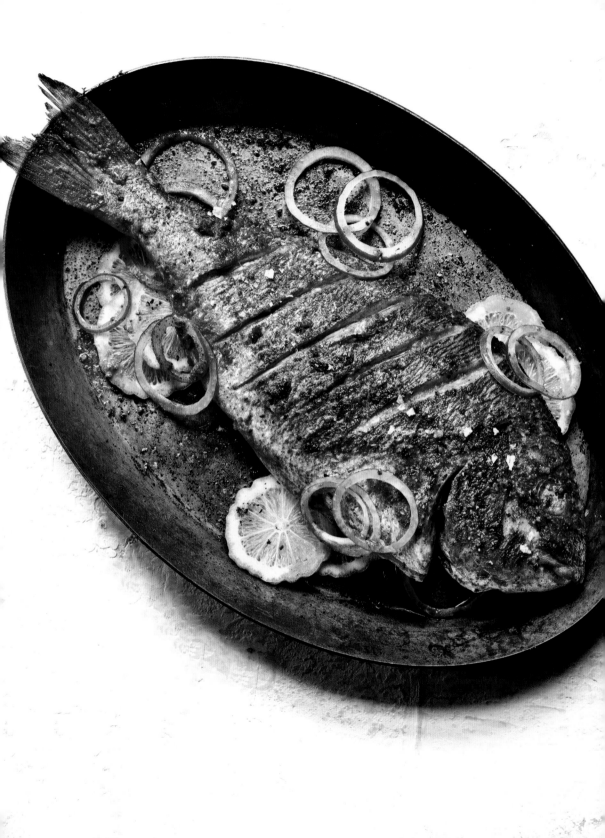

PAN-SEARED SEA BREAM

SERVES 2

Pan-seared fish like sea bream and bass are food heaven for me, especially when the skin is extra crispy. This is normally done with substantially more oil and by scraping the excess moisture from the skin before frying. Preparing the skin so that it is dry for frying is explained below. I suggest using a non-stick frying pan for this low-calorie version so that the skin doesn't stick to the pan.

PREP TIME: 10 MINS
COOKING TIME: 10 MINS

2 sea bream, scaled and cleaned
2 tbsp garlic and ginger paste
1 tsp garam masala (see page 146)
1 tsp ground coriander
½ tsp ground turmeric
3 generous tsp Kashmiri chilli powder
½ tsp salt, plus more to taste
3 tbsp malt vinegar or coconut vinegar
2 tbsp rapeseed (canola) oil
Sliced red onion rings, to serve
Lemon slices, to serve

Press a sharp knife at a 45-degree angle onto the fish just after the head and scrape the skin with it right down to the tail. When you do this, you will notice that a lot of excess moisture is on your knife. Dry it off with paper towel, then repeat on both sides of the fish as many times as necessary until the skin is really dry to the touch. This will help ensure the skin is nice and crispy once fried. Make shallow slits on each side of the fish about 2.5cm (1 inch) apart.

In a bowl, mix all the remaining ingredients up to and including the vinegar together to make the marinade. If you aren't sure about the spiciness, I recommend adding less chilli powder than suggested, or if you like your food spicy hot, add a little more. The more chilli you use, the nicer the finished dish will look. Rub the marinade all over the fish. You are now ready to fry but you could leave the marinade on for about 20 minutes if that is more convenient.

When ready to cook, heat the oil in a frying pan over a medium–high heat. Cook the fish for about 5 minutes on each side, or until the skin is crispy and the fish is just cooked through. Serve garnished with sliced red onion rings and lemon slices.

PANEER ACHARI CURRY
SERVES 4

The word 'achari' refers to the pickling spices used in this recipe. They make the sauce amazing. It is important to add the paneer just at the end of cooking and simmer it in the sauce until it is heated through and mouth-wateringly soft. I find paneer to be the perfect meat substitute. It's filling and not too high in calories. A little goes a long way.

PREP TIME: 10 MINS
COOKING TIME: 15 MINS

2 green chillies, roughly chopped
2 tsp coriander seeds
1 tbsp fennel seeds
2 tsp cumin seeds
½ tsp fenugreek seeds
400g (14oz) chopped tomatoes
1 red (bell) pepper, roughly chopped
1 tbsp mustard oil or rapeseed (canola) oil
1 tbsp black mustard seeds
2 onions, finely chopped
1 tbsp garlic and ginger paste
½ tsp ground turmeric
1 tsp chilli powder
Salt, to taste
1 tsp sugar or sugar substitute, to taste
250g (1 cup) fat-free plain yoghurt
200g (7oz) paneer, cubed
3 tbsp finely chopped coriander (cilantro), to garnish
5cm (2-inch) piece of ginger, peeled and cut into matchsticks, to garnish
Juice of 1 lemon

Heat a dry frying pan over a medium–high heat and toast the green chillies and whole spices until fragrant and warm to the touch. Allow to cool, then grind to a fine powder using a spice grinder or pestle and mortar. Set aside. Place the tomatoes and red (bell) pepper in a blender and blend to a smooth purée.

Heat the oil in a large frying pan over a medium–high heat until visibly hot. Add the mustard seeds and when they begin to pop (after about 30 seconds), add the onions and fry for about 5 minutes until soft, lightly browned and translucent. If it looks like the onions are sticking to the pan, reduce the heat to medium.

Add the garlic and ginger paste and fry for about 30 seconds while stirring into the onion mixture. Working on a medium heat, stir in the ground turmeric and chilli powder and continue frying for about 30 seconds, then mix in the puréed pepper and tomato. Continue cooking until the sauce is quite thick. Add salt and sugar to taste, then reduce the heat to low.

Stir in the yoghurt, 1 tablespoon at a time – if you add it too quickly it will curdle. Add about 70ml (¼ cup) water to thin the sauce, then cover and simmer for about 3 minutes, or until you are happy with the consistency.

Add the paneer to the sauce and stir well to combine. Cook on a low heat for about 3 minutes until the paneer is heated through – you don't want to cook the paneer too long or it will fall apart. To serve, season with salt and garnish with the coriander, ginger and a squeeze of lemon juice.

ALOO GOBI
SERVES 2

With this recipe I wanted to demonstrate the low-sodium, low-fat onion caramelization method on page 151. No need to flip pages, we are going to do it all right here. Aloo gobi, when done correctly, can be amazing, but it is often a bit mushy. Not with this recipe – you will get perfect results every time. The key is in first cooking the potatoes and cauliflower separately, then finishing the dish with everything cooked together. This takes a bit more time, but the end result warrants it. A large saucepan with a lid is essential, non-stick is even better.

PREP TIME: 10 MINS
COOKING TIME: 20 MINS,
OR UNTIL TENDER

175g (6oz) potatoes, cut into
    4cm (1½-inch) cubes
2 tbsp rapeseed (canola) oil
250g (9oz) large cauliflower
    florets, sliced in half so that
    the stalks are thin
¼ cinnamon stick
1 tsp cumin seeds
5 black peppercorns
2 cloves
1 large onion, finely chopped
1 tbsp garlic and ginger paste
1–2 green bird's eye chillies, cut
    into rings
1 large or 2 medium tomatoes,
    diced
½ tsp ground turmeric
½ tsp Kashmiri chilli powder
½ tsp ground coriander
Salt and freshly ground black
    pepper, to taste
Juice of 1 lime
3 tbsp finely chopped coriander
    (cilantro)

Place the potatoes in a bowl of water for about 10 minutes. As a guide, these should be just slightly smaller than the cauliflower florets. Soaking the potatoes in water will get rid of any excess starch and also stop them from discolouring.

Meanwhile, heat 1 tablespoon of the oil in a frying pan over a low–medium heat. The pan should be large enough to hold all the cauliflower florets in one layer. Move the florets around in the pan until brown marks begin to appear, then transfer to a bowl. In what remains of the oil in the pan, do the same with the potatoes – you just want to move them around for about 3 minutes until they look lightly browned. If it looks like they are sticking to the pan, you can add a drop of water. Transfer to the bowl with the cauliflower.

Add the remaining oil to the pan. When hot, add the whole spices and infuse them in the oil for about 30 seconds. Add the onion and fry over a low–medium heat for about 20 minutes until browned and caramelized – a pinch of salt will help the process. If needed, add a drop of water, but not too much as you want to caramelize the onion, not boil it. When nicely browned, stir in the garlic and ginger paste and chillies and fry for about 30 seconds, then stir in the tomatoes, ground spices, seared cauliflower and potatoes.

Stir well and add a little water if you prefer a thinner sauce. Cover the pan and simmer on a low–medium heat for 5 minutes, or until the potatoes and cauliflower are cooked to your liking. Season with salt and black pepper and squeeze the lime juice over the top. Serve, garnished with the coriander.

BUTTERNUT SQUASH CURRY
SERVES 4

This hearty squash curry is delicious served over rice or scooped up with masala rotis (see page 122). In the photograph I have served it with dry-fried papadams, using the same method used in the papad cone recipe on page 16. This is common in India, where they enjoy lots of different textures in a meal. In the UK we tend to see papadams only as starters, but their crispy texture and flavour goes so well with the soft cooked squash. Sometimes I cook this just as the recipe is and then I purée any leftovers for a smoother and creamier variation. The blended purée is also amazing as a garnish for seafood, such as the grilled tuna on page 112. I like to serve this with the pickled pearl onions on page 136 and perhaps a good raita like the coriander and chilli raita, also on page 136.

PREP TIME: 10 MINS
COOKING TIME: 20 MINS

1½ tbsp rapeseed (canola) oil
1 tsp black mustard seeds
1 tsp cumin seeds
10 fresh or frozen curry leaves
1 red onion, finely chopped
2 green chillies, finely chopped
    (more or less, to taste)
1½ tbsp garlic and ginger paste
½ tsp ground turmeric
1 tsp chilli powder (more or less,
    to taste)
1 tsp ground coriander
1 medium butternut squash,
    peeled, seeded and cut into
    1.5cm (½-inch) cubes
    (roughly 700g/1lb 9oz
    prepared weight)
400ml (scant 1¾ cups) low-fat
    coconut milk
200g (7oz) fresh or frozen peas
Salt, to taste
½ tsp garam masala (see page
    146)
3 tbsp finely chopped coriander
    (cilantro)

Heat the oil in a large frying pan or wok over a high heat until visibly hot. Add the mustard seeds and when they begin to crackle (after about 30 seconds), reduce the heat to medium–high and toss in the cumin seeds and curry leaves. Let these flavours infuse into the oil for about 30 seconds. Stir in the onion and fry for about 5 minutes until soft and translucent. Add the green chillies and garlic and ginger paste and stir it all up to combine. Fry this base masala for about 1 minute, then stir in the ground spices, followed by the squash and fry for about 5 minutes, or until the squash is about half cooked through.

Add the coconut milk and the peas and cover the pan. Simmer for about 5 minutes until the squash is soft and the peas are cooked through. You might need to add a little water, but remember that this is a dry curry, so don't add too much unless you prefer a soupier curry, which is fine. Season with salt and garnish with the garam masala and coriander.

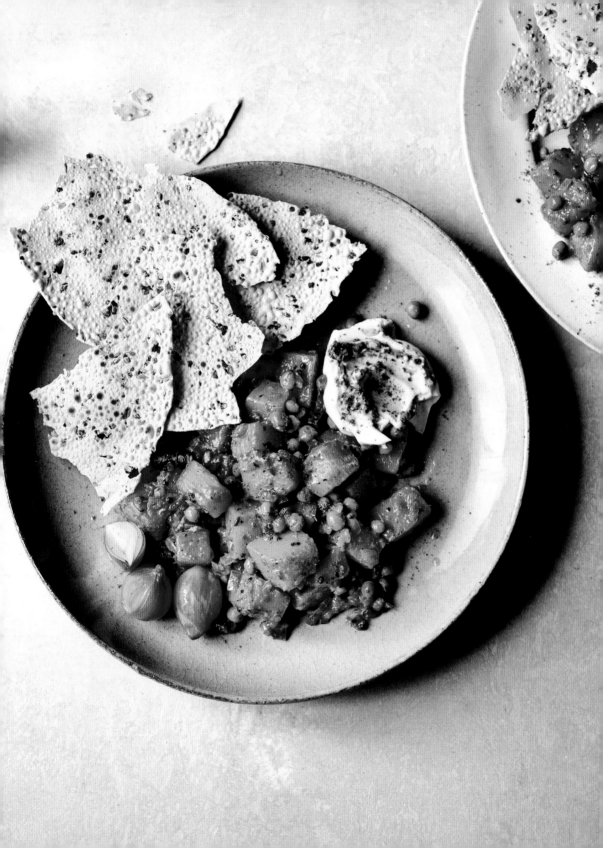

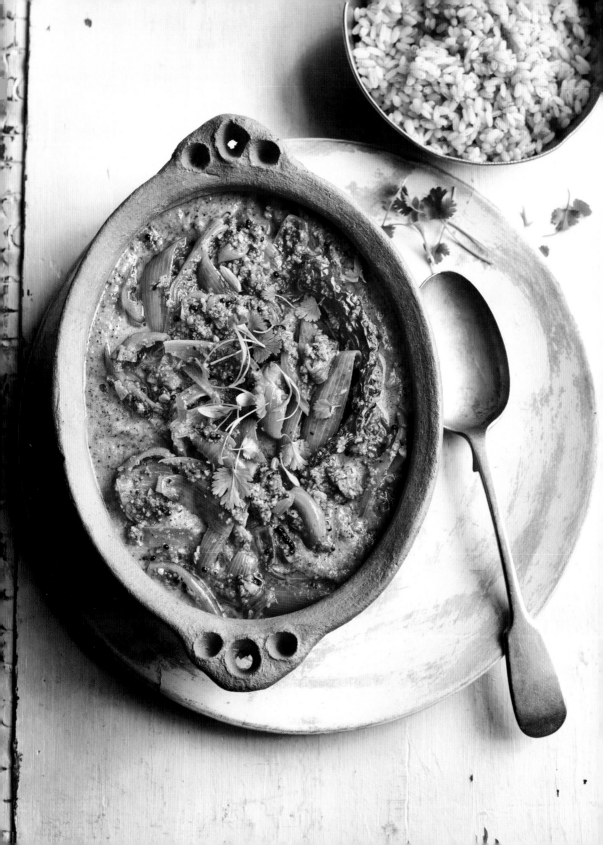

SHALLOT CURRY

SERVES 4

This has to be one of my favourite veggie curries. It is so good drizzled over matta rice (see page 123). The first time I tried this recipe, it was brought to our table boiling hot and very smooth at a restaurant in Alleppey, Kerala. Both my wife and I loved it and ordered the shallot curry (ulli theeyal) a few more times at restaurants around Kerala, but it was never as good as the first time. A lot of chefs cook this curry leaving the shallots whole, but I prefer them blended. Try it both ways to see which you prefer – smooth or chunky? In the photograph opposite, I blended the curry but left a few shallots whole for a garnish.

PREP TIME: 20 MINS
COOKING TIME: 20 MINS

1 golf ball-sized piece of
    tamarind or 1 tsp tamarind
    paste (see page 149) or
    concentrate
600ml (2½ cups) hot water

FOR THE PASTE
¼ tsp fenugreek seeds
1 tsp cumin seeds
1 tsp whole black peppercorns
2 tsp coriander seeds
1 tsp rapeseed (canola) oil
200g (7oz) grated coconut

FOR THE SAUCE
2 tbsp rapeseed (canola) oil or
    coconut oil
1 tsp black mustard seeds
½ tsp cumin seeds
¼ tsp fenugreek seeds
2 dried red Kashmiri chillies
10 fresh or frozen curry leaves
20 shallots, peeled and cut into
    about three pieces
5 garlic cloves, finely chopped
¼ tsp ground turmeric
2 tsp ground coriander
2 tsp ground cumin
1–2 tsp Kashmiri chilli powder
Salt, to taste
Coriander (cilantro), to garnish

Place the tamarind in a bowl and cover with the hot water. When cool enough to handle, squeeze the tamarind into the water and run it through a fine-mesh sieve into another bowl, discarding any pulp.

To make the paste, heat a dry frying pan over a medium–high heat and toast the fenugreek seeds, cumin seeds, peppercorns and coriander seeds for about 30 seconds until fragrant and warm to the touch. Transfer to a plate to cool. Heat the oil in the same pan over a low heat and fry the coconut until golden brown. Transfer the coconut and toasted spices to a spice grinder or pestle and mortar and add just enough water to grind into a smooth paste. Set aside.

Now make the sauce. Heat the oil in a large pot – preferably a clay pot if you have one – over a medium–high heat until visibly hot. Add the black mustard seeds and when they begin to pop (after about 30 seconds), reduce the heat to medium and add the cumin seeds, fenugreek seeds, dried chillies and curry leaves. Give this all a good stir and allow the spices to infuse into the oil for about 30 seconds, then add the shallots. Sauté, stirring often until the shallots begin to turn translucent; this should take about 5 minutes. Now stir in the garlic and all the ground spices and continue frying for 2 minutes.

Add the ground coconut/spice paste and sauté for a further 3 minutes. Pour in the tamarind water and cook for about 5 minutes until the sauce thickens and the oil floats to the top. You could skim this off if you like, but I usually leave it in. Check for seasoning and add salt if needed. Serve as is or blend the curry until smooth – my favourite way to have it.

Just before serving, garnish with the coriander.

BABY SWEETCORN & CHILLI STIR-FRY

SERVES 4

This is a dry curry that could be served as a side or main. If serving as a main, I recommend serving this with a good dhal and/or chapattis and your choice of raitas. It is also nice with hot sauce.

PREP TIME: 5 MINS
COOKING TIME: 15–20
MINS

2 tbsp rapeseed (canola) oil
1 tsp cumin seeds
5 fresh or frozen curry leaves
   (optional)
2 medium onions, finely
   chopped
400g (2 generous cups) baby
   sweetcorn, cut into small
   pieces
1–3 green bird's eye chillies,
   finely chopped
1 small red (bell) pepper, roughly
   chopped
1 tsp Kashmiri chilli powder
½ tsp ground turmeric
½ tsp garam masala (see page
   146) or bafat curry powder for
   a spicier result (see page 149)
Salt and freshly ground black
   pepper, to taste
2 tbsp chopped coriander
   (cilantro), to garnish

Heat the oil in a large frying pan over a medium–high heat until visibly hot. Add the cumin seeds and curry leaves (if using) and temper them in the oil for about 30 seconds. Add the onions and fry for about 5 minutes until soft and translucent.

Now add the baby sweetcorn, chillies, red pepper, chilli powder, ground turmeric and garam masala or bafat curry powder. Stir well to coat the corn with the spice and onion mixture and continue cooking for 15–20 minutes, stirring regularly until the corn is cooked through and the onions are sweet and browned. Season with salt and black pepper and garnish with the coriander before serving.

BAKED STUFFED RAVA AUBERGINES

SERVES 2

This one is great served as a vegetarian main course or as a starter to serve four. I have tried this with fine and coarse semolina and prefer the coarse finish, but my wife likes fine better. Therefore, that is, of course, exactly how I usually make this one!

PREP TIME: 15 MINS
COOKING TIME: 15 MINS

1 large aubergine (eggplant), cut into four 2.5cm (1-inch) slices from the middle

FOR THE STUFFING
Salt, to taste
2 potatoes, peeled and cut into small cubes
2 tsp coconut oil or rapeseed (canola) oil
1 tsp black mustard seeds
5 fresh or frozen curry leaves
1 tsp asafoetida
1 generous tbsp garlic and ginger paste
1 green chilli, finely chopped
1 tbsp cumin seeds
50g (¼ cup) cauliflower
1 medium carrot (about 50g/1¾oz), peeled and grated
½ tsp ground turmeric
1 tsp Kashmiri chilli powder
2 tbsp fine semolina
Cooking spray or rapeseed (canola) oil, for greasing
Hot sauce of choice or raita(s), to serve
3 tbsp finely chopped coriander (cilantro)

Remove the pulp in the middle of the aubergine (eggplant) by carving out a circle, but leaving about 1cm (½ inch) of aubergine around the border. You can keep the aubergine pulp for other uses, such my vegetable biryani on page 78.

Meanwhile, make the stuffing. Bring a saucepan of lightly salted water to a boil and add the potatoes. Simmer for about 10 minutes, or until the potatoes are fork tender. Drain and lightly mash the potatoes with a fork.

Heat the oil in a frying pan over a high heat until visibly hot. Add the mustard seeds and when they begin to crackle (after about 30 seconds), reduce the heat to medium–high and add the curry leaves, asafoetida, garlic and ginger paste, green chilli and cumin seeds and temper in the oil for about 30 seconds.

Add the cauliflower, mashed potatoes and carrot, then stir in the ground turmeric and chilli powder and fry over a low heat for about 10 minutes. If it looks like the veggies are sticking to the pan, add a drop of water. Set aside to cool slightly. Rinse the aubergine rings and wipe dry with paper towel. Spoon the stuffing into the holes in the aubergines. Pour the semolina on a plate and carefully coat the stuffed aubergines in it.

Preheat the oven to 220°C (425°F/Gas 7). Line a baking tray with greaseproof (waxed) paper and lightly spray it with cooking spray or grease it with oil. Place the stuffed aubergines on the tray and either brush or spray them lightly with cooking spray or oil too. Bake for about 20 minutes, or until nicely browned. Serve immediately with the hot sauce of your choice or a raita or two, and garnish with the coriander.

NOTE
Polenta can be substituted for the semolina to make this gluten free. Do also note that some brands of asafoetida contain gluten, so do check the packaging.

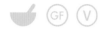

VEGETABLE & PANEER DUM BIRYANI

SERVES 8

To make a fragrant biryani in this way, you need a pot with a very tight-fitting lid. If you don't have one, cover the pot tightly with foil, then put the lid on top. This is a delicious biryani that is great served on special occasions. Lift the lid at the table and enjoy the fantastic aroma as the steam fills the room.

PREP TIME: 20 MINS, PLUS SOAKING TIME
COOKING TIME: 30 MINS

370g (2 cups) basmati rice
4 star anise
10 black peppercorns
1 cinnamon stick
1 tsp salt

FOR THE SAUCE

2 tbsp ghee
2 star anise
1 cinnamon stick
1 tsp cumin seeds
3 cloves
1 onion, finely chopped
2 tbsp garlic and ginger paste
50g (1¾oz) each of broccoli florets and aubergine (cut into small cubes), carrot (roughly chopped), baby potatoes (cut into thirds), peas and green beans (cut into small pieces)
250g (1 cup) low-fat Greek yoghurt
½ tsp ground turmeric
2 tsp Kashmiri chilli powder (more or less, to taste)
1 tbsp garam masala (see page 146)
200g (7oz) paneer, cut into small cubes
Salt and freshly ground black pepper, to taste
A good pinch of saffron
125ml (½ cup) hand-hot low-fat milk
20g (¾oz) coriander (cilantro), finely chopped
20g (¾oz) mint, finely chopped
1 onion, sliced and caramelized (optional, see page 151)

Place the rice in a large bowl and cover with water. Swirl it around in the water until it becomes cloudy, then drain. Repeat this process until the water runs almost clear. Cover the rice with water again and soak for 30 minutes, then drain.

Bring 1½ litres (6 cups) of water to the boil with the star anise, black peppercorns, cinnamon stick and salt and tip in the soaked rice. Simmer the rice for about 6 minutes until it is almost cooked through but still a bit hard. Drain and rinse under cold water. Set aside.

Now make the sauce. Melt 1 tablespoon of the ghee in a large saucepan that is just big enough to hold the rice and sauce. Toss in the star anise, cinnamon stick, cumin seeds and cloves and let these spices infuse into the ghee for about 30 seconds. Stir in the onion and fry for about 5 minutes until soft and translucent, then add the garlic and ginger paste. Stir it all up to combine and cook out the rawness of the garlic and ginger for about 30 seconds.

Add the vegetables and fry for about 3 minutes, then add the yoghurt, turmeric, chilli powder and garam masala. Cook for another minute, then stir the paneer into the sauce. Remove from the heat and season with salt and black pepper. Transfer two-thirds of the sauce to a bowl.

In a cup, stir the saffron into the warmed milk. Add the remaining tablespoon of ghee to the saffron/milk mixture. Now cover the remaining sauce in the pot with one-third of the rice and top with some of the coriander and mint, some low-fat caramelized onions (if using) and drizzle with one-third of the saffron/milk mixture. Repeat with two more layers. Place the lid back on the pot and steam over a low–medium heat for a further 20 minutes. To serve, stir it all up at the table and dig in.

NOTE

This biryani is delicious and moist just as it is. However, I can highly recommend serving it with my low-calorie pickled pearl onions and/or cucumber raita on page 136.

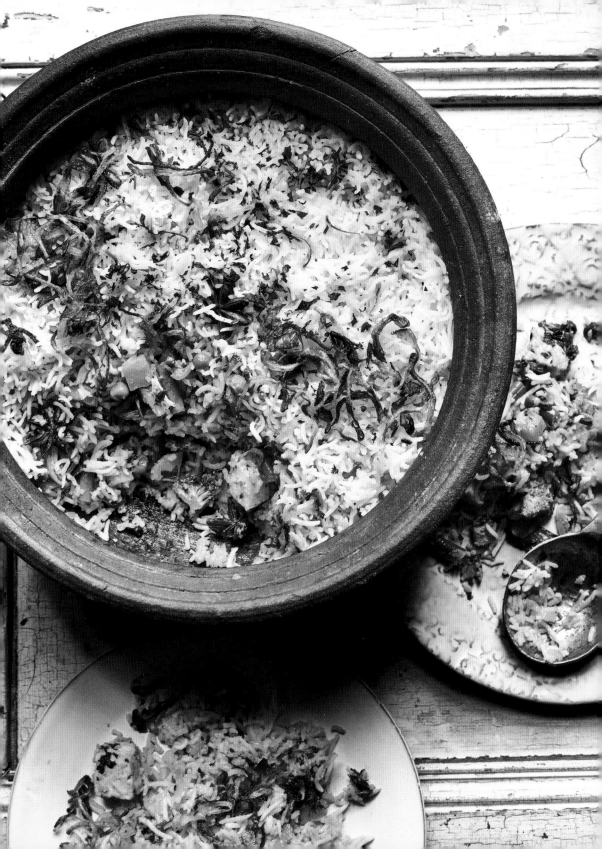

LIGHT BRITISH CURRY-HOUSE-STYLE CURRIES

You know how when you go to a curry house and each of the traditional curries is offered with meat, seafood and vegetable options? Well that is what I have on offer for you here too. You see, the magic of the dish is in the sauce. What you serve in that sauce is up to you. I have given some popular options for each of the curries in this chapter, but feel free to tailor the recipes to your own dietary wishes.

On page 145 I feature a recipe for a lamb or chicken soup, which can also be made vegetarian. Make and enjoy the soup or use the idea behind the recipe to prepare pre-cooked meat, vegetables and stock to go into your curries.

THE BASE SAUCE

The curry-house base sauce or gravy is essential to achieving that British curry-house flavour and texture. I featured many recipes that used a base sauce in my first two cookbooks. For the most part, people enjoyed preparing the base sauce and loved the fact that once it was made, they could cook their favourite curries in 10 minutes or less. There were a few, however, who thought it was a step too far as it had to be made before they could get started.

In this book I have developed a light version of the base sauce that is just as good as the full-fat version. This base sauce serves two purposes: not only can it be used, as most curry-house chefs do, to cook the now world-famous British curries, it also offers a great way of cooking up a curry with a lot less fat and no loss of flavour.

It is my hope that, even if you don't like the idea of making a base sauce ahead of the main recipe, you will have a go at making the super-easy, quick, low-fat one featured on the following page. Not only will you be able to make light curry-house-style curries that can compete with any full-fat versions, you will see from the recipe that it's really good for you too! It freezes well, so no procrastinating! This fresh and smooth vegetable base sauce is the beginning of convenience food at its best.

BASE SAUCE SUBSTITUTE

The base sauce is really just the liquid required to cook the curry. In authentic Indian cooking, a base masala of ingredients like oil, onions, garlic, ginger, tomatoes and water are used to make the sauce, along with other spices and ingredients. Use more authentic cooking methods and you will get a more authentic-textured curry that is different to British curry-house-style curries but still very good. To demonstrate how you can make the following curries without a base sauce, I have done just that with my Kashmiri chicken recipe on page 95. If you would like to use a base sauce in that recipe instead, forget frying up that base masala and use about 300ml (1¼ cups) of prepared light base sauce.

PRE-COOKED INGREDIENTS

From tandoori chicken to vegetable kebabs, keema and base sauce, British Indian restaurant (BIR) cooking is all about convenience and getting in those additional layers of flavour. Using grilled tandoori chicken rather than raw chicken in your chicken tikka masala sauce will give the sauce a more complex flavour. The prep does take a little longer, but it's well worth the extra time. You can, of course, use raw chicken, and though the sauce will still taste amazing, it will lack the depth of flavour you'd get using grilled chicken.

I would like to encourage you to make these recipes the way you want. If you don't have time to marinate and grill tandoori chicken or meat for a recipe, just cook it from raw or purchase some tandoori chicken from the supermarket. You might need to add more liquid if cooking from raw. Red meat like beef and lamb benefit from pre-cooking as they take longer to cook and become tender. If a quick, tasty takeaway-style meal is what you desire, you will get that in the following recipes. If you are looking for a one-pot, minimal-fuss meal, you might like to try one of the authentic Indian curries (see pages 32–79) instead.

LOW-CALORIE BASE CURRY SAUCE

SERVES 14–16; MAKES ABOUT 3 LITRES (13 CUPS)

The base sauce is the magical ingredient behind all good curry-house curries. It is bland because it has to be as it's used in everything from the mildest korma up to the spiciest phal. It is essentially a smooth onion stock with a few other healthy ingredients thrown into the mix.

PREP TIME: 20 MINS
COOKING TIME: 1¼ HOURS

1kg (2lb 4oz/about 7) onions
2 tbsp rapeseed (canola) oil
½ teaspoon salt
1 litre (4½ cups) water, or
    chicken or vegetable stock
100g (3½oz) carrots, peeled and
    chopped
60g (2oz) cabbage, chopped
½ red (bell) pepper, diced
½ green (bell) pepper, diced
8 garlic cloves
5cm (2-inch) piece of ginger,
    peeled and roughly chopped
200g (7oz) tinned (canned)
    chopped tomatoes
1½ tbsp garam masala (see page
    146)
1½ tbsp ground cumin
1½ tbsp ground coriander
1½ tbsp paprika
1 tbsp ground fenugreek
½ tbsp ground turmeric

Finely slice the onions by hand or in a food processor. Heat the oil in a large stockpot and fry the onions for about 5 minutes until soft and fragrant, stirring well until evenly coated in the oil. Add all the ingredients up to and including the tomatoes. Cover the pot and simmer over a medium heat for about 1 hour. The vegetables will become soft and the stock should reduce by about half, but this can vary. How much it reduces down is not important at this stage. Add the ground spices and simmer for a further 5 minutes.

Using a stick blender or worktop blender, blend until very smooth – you shouldn't see any chunks. If you are thinking about freezing some of the sauce, now is the perfect time to do so.

To use this in your curries, you need to stir in enough water or unsalted stock until the sauce is the same consistency as single cream – so very runny! I normally just add water, which is how most restaurant chefs make their base stocks, but if I know I will be using the base for a specific curry, I substitute unsalted stock instead, which adds extra flavour. The stock produced making the chicken/lamb stock soup on page 145 – minus the chillies, chilli powder and coconut – works really well. I would use chicken stock for a chicken curry, and lamb stock for a lamb curry. This is all optional, however, as the stock made with water will work in any curry.

This base sauce will keep in the fridge for about a week and it can be frozen for up to four months.

TIP

If you are freezing any of the base sauce, do it before adding the additional water/stock at the end. This will save freezer space. Then just defrost it, heat it up and add enough water or stock until the sauce is the same consistency as single cream.

CHICKEN & CHICKPEA CURRY

SERVES 2

Here's one I made up one evening when I needed to use up some ingredients. This is really just a normal chicken curry like those seen on so many curry house menus with some chickpeas thrown in. I love chickpeas in a curry and they went really well with this mildly spiced combo. This is great with the tandoori chicken tikka on page 102, but if you don't have any to hand you can cut some raw chicken into small, bite-sized pieces and let it cook through in the sauce.

PREP TIME: 5 MINS, PLUS
PRE-COOKED INGREDIENT
TIME
COOKING TIME: 10 MINS

1 tbsp rapeseed (canola) oil
½ onion, finely chopped
2 tsp garlic and ginger paste
70ml (¼ cup) tomato purée (see page 146)
1 tsp paprika or chilli powder
1 tbsp mixed powder (see page 150) or curry powder
300ml (1¼ cups) low-calorie base curry sauce (see page 82), heated
400g (14oz) tinned (canned) chickpeas, drained (about 250g/9oz drained weight)
125g (4½oz) skinless chicken breast cut into bite-sized pieces or tandoori chicken tikka (see page 102)
About 70ml (¼ cup) unsalted chicken stock or meat juices from the tandoori chicken (optional)
½ tsp dried fenugreek leaves (kasoori methi)
½ tsp garam masala (see page 146)
Juice of ½ lemon
Salt, to taste
2 tbsp finely chopped coriander (cilantro), to garnish
2.5cm (1-inch) piece of ginger, peeled and julienned

Heat the oil in a frying pan over a medium–high heat until hot. Fry the onion for about 3 minutes until it becomes translucent and soft. Stir in the garlic and ginger paste and fry for 30 seconds or so.

Add the tomato purée and let it bubble for about 1 minute. Stir in the paprika or chilli powder and the mixed powder or curry powder, then pour in about 125ml (½ cup) of the base curry sauce. Bring to a simmer without stirring, unless it is obviously sticking. If any of the sauce caramelizes to the sides of the pan, stir it in.

Add the chickpeas and chicken, along with the rest of the sauce. If using tandoori chicken and you have any meat juices from the cooking, add a little of this for extra flavour. Alternatively you could add a little unsalted chicken stock if you wish.

Simmer for a further 5 minutes, or until the chicken is cooked through and you are happy with the consistency of the sauce. When cooking chicken from raw, you may need to add a splash more base stock or chicken stock to cook it through.

To finish, sprinkle in the dried fenugreek leaves (kasoori methi), rubbing the leaves between your fingers to release their flavour, then sprinkle on the garam masala, and squeeze over the lemon juice. Check for seasoning and add salt if necessary. Garnish with the coriander and ginger and serve.

CHICKEN TIKKA MASALA
SERVES 2

In my opinion, chicken tikka masala has to be made with tandoori-style chicken (see page 102). This brings with in another layer of flavour that really complements this curry. Chicken tikka masala is well known for being buttery, sweet and creamy. Here, the buttery flavour is achieved with a large dose of ground almonds and just enough sugar is used to make it mildly sweet. A good artificial sweetener could be added to taste instead with good results. Whisked fat-free yoghurt makes the curry incredibly creamy without all the fat of cream.

PREP TIME: 10 MINS, PLUS
PRE-COOKED INGREDIENT
TIME
COOKING TIME: 10 MINS

1 tbsp rapeseed (canola) oil or coconut oil
2 tsp garlic and ginger paste
2 tbsp ground almonds
2 tbsp coconut flour
2 tsp mixed powder (see page 150) or curry powder
1½ tbsp tandoori masala (see page 148)
1 tsp sweet paprika
5 tbsp tomato purée (see page 146)
350ml (1½ cups) low-calorie base curry sauce (see page 82), heated
200g (7oz) tandoori chicken tikka (see page 102) or raw chicken breast, cut into bite-sized pieces
1 tbsp sugar or artificial sweetener of choice (or to taste) (optional)
80ml (⅓ cup) fat-free plain yoghurt
1 tsp red food colouring powder (optional)
1½ tsp lemon juice
2 tbsp finely chopped coriander (cilantro)
1 tsp dried fenugreek leaves (kasoori methi)
½ tsp garam masala (see page 146)
Salt, to taste
Coriander (cilantro), to garnish

Heat the oil in a Balti pan or frying pan over a medium–high heat. When hot, add the garlic and ginger paste and sizzle for about 30 seconds. Add the ground almonds and coconut flour and fry for a further 20 seconds while stirring constantly. The pan will look quite dry as the almonds and coconut soak up the oil. Stir in the remaining spices, then add the tomato purée and the base sauce.

Increase the heat to high and allow the sauce to come to a rolling simmer. Stir in the tandoori chicken and heat through for a few minutes. If using raw chicken, it will need about 5 minutes' simmering in the sauce to cook it through.

Once the meat is heated/cooked through, reduce the heat to medium–high and stir in sugar (if using). Now add the yoghurt, one tablespoon at a time. If using food colouring, stir it in now, then squeeze in the lemon juice and add the coriander.

To finish, add the dried fenugreek leaves (kasoori methi), rubbing the leaves between your fingers to help bring out their flavour. Top with the garam masala, season with salt to taste and garnish with coriander.

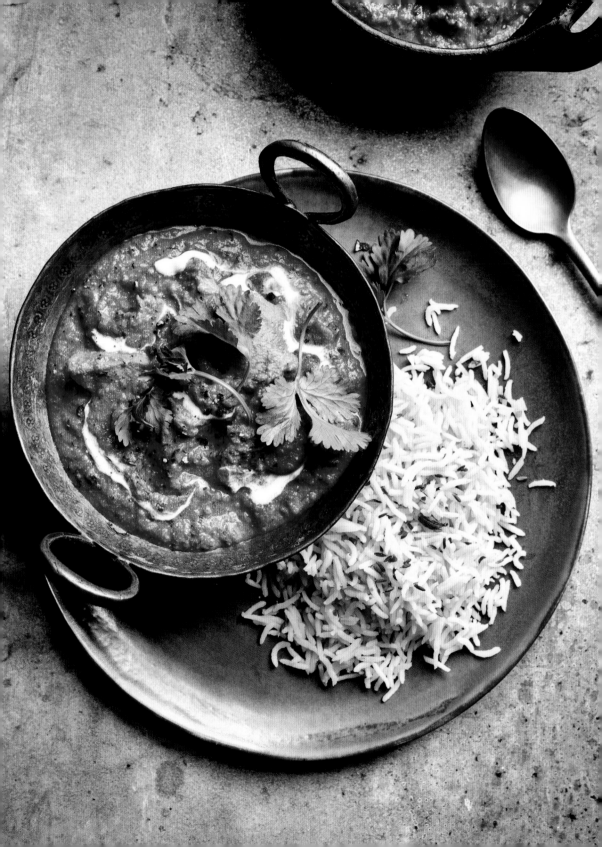

CHICKEN JALFREZI
SERVES 2

Chicken jalfrezi is one of the most ordered curries at curry houses all over the UK. Like so many of these curries that are usually a bit on the heavy side, chicken jalfrezi can easily made low fat without losing that fantastic flavour. Cooking oil and ghee are used a lot in curry-house-style curries because they taste great and also make the cooking process a bit easier. Therefore, when cooking with less oil, you really need to watch it! I usually add the ingredients in a different order too, as I've done below, to lessen the chance of burning the spices, which could make the curry rather bitter and not very nice. Follow these instructions and you will end up with a curry-house-style chicken jalfrezi that is right up there with the best. Believe me... you won't miss the extra fat.

PREP TIME: 10 MINS, PLUS
PRE-COOKED INGREDIENT
TIME
COOKING TIME: 10 MINS

1 tbsp rapeseed (canola) oil or
    coconut oil
5 fresh or frozen curry leaves
½ red (bell) pepper, thinly sliced
½ green (bell) pepper, thinly
    sliced
1 medium onion, thinly sliced
2 green chillies, cut into rings
2 spring onions (scallions),
    thinly sliced
10 cherry tomatoes, halved
1 tbsp garlic and ginger paste
70ml (¼ cup) tomato purée (see
    page 146)
1 generous tbsp mixed powder
    (see page 150) or curry
    powder
½ tsp chilli powder (more or
    less, to taste)
300ml (1¼ cups) low-calorie
    base curry sauce (see page 82)
200g (7oz) tandoori chicken
    tikka (see page 102)
Salt, to taste
2 tbsp chopped coriander
    (cilantro)

Heat the oil in a Balti pan or frying pan over a medium–high heat. Stir in the curry leaves, followed immediately by the red and green peppers, onion, chillies and spring onions and stir so that the veggies are completely coated with the oil. Fry for about 2 minutes, then add half the cherry tomatoes and the garlic and ginger paste. Fry for another minute, then add the tomato purée, stirring well to combine.

Add the spices and the base curry sauce. Let the sauce simmer for 3–5 minutes until you are happy with the consistency, then add the tandoori chicken tikka. You could add raw chicken, but you might need to add a little more base sauce or water to help it cook through. When the chicken is almost heated through (or if using raw chicken, cooked through – after about 5 minutes), stir in the remaining cherry tomatoes. Continue to cook for about 2 minutes until the tomatoes are heated through but remain fresh looking. Season with salt and garnish with the coriander.

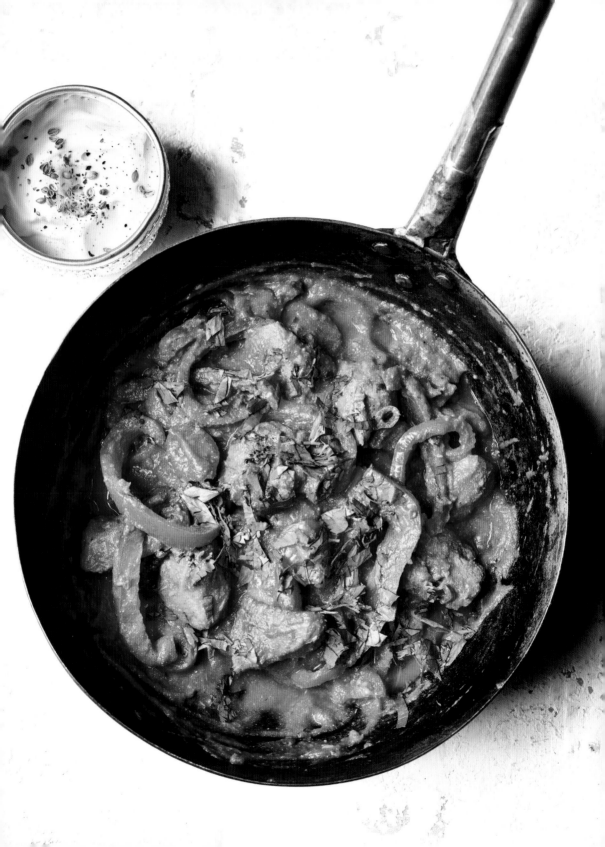

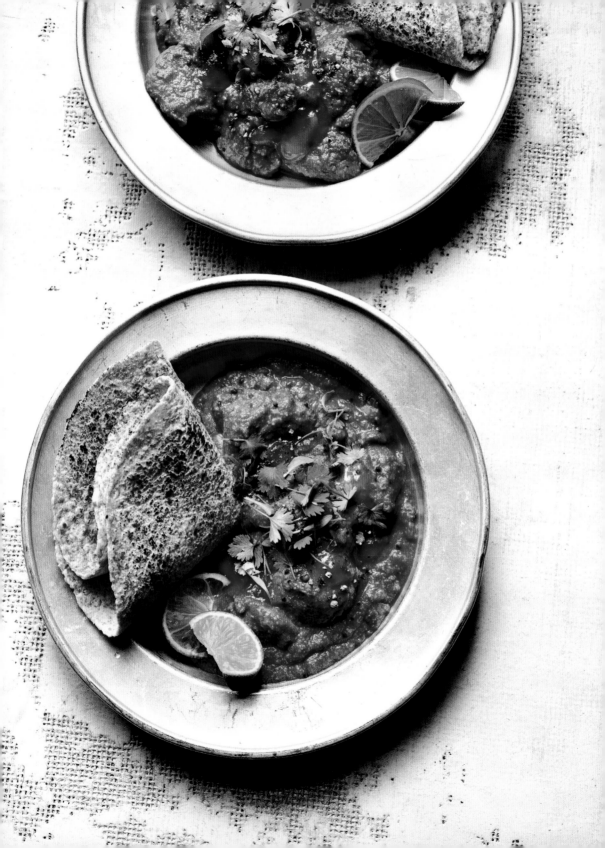

CHICKEN CEYLON
SERVES 2

This recipe might have a lot of ingredients, but get them lined up and weighed out before you start and the recipe is a breeze. I like to serve this with warm chapattis.

PREP TIME: 10 MINS, PLUS
PRE-COOKED INGREDIENT
TIME
COOKING TIME: 10 MINS

1 tbsp coconut oil or rapeseed (canola) oil
½ tsp black mustard seeds
1 star anise
2 green cardamom pods, smashed
½ cinnamon stick
5 fresh or frozen curry leaves
2 tsp garlic and ginger paste
1–2 green bird's-eye chillies, finely chopped
2 tbsp coconut flour
1½ tbsp finely chopped coriander (cilantro) stalks
70ml (¼ cup) tomato purée (see page 146)
300ml (1¼ cups) low-calorie base curry sauce (see page 82), heated
175ml (¾ cup) light coconut milk
½ tsp Kashmiri chilli powder
2 tsp mixed powder (see page 150) or curry powder
1 tbsp tandoori masala (see page 148)
1 tsp freshly ground black pepper
200g (7oz) tandoori chicken tikka (see page 102) or chicken breast, cut into bite-sized pieces
½ tsp dried fenugreek leaves (kasoori methi)
2 tsp smooth mango chutney
Juice of 1 lime
½ tsp garam masala (see page 146)
Salt, to taste
1 tbsp chopped coriander (cilantro), to garnish

Heat the oil in a Balti pan or frying pan over a medium–high heat. When visibly hot, add the mustard seeds. When they begin to crackle (after about 30 seconds), add the star anise, cardamom pods, cinnamon and curry leaves and temper them in the oil for about 20 seconds. Stir in the garlic and ginger paste and the green chillies and fry for a further 20 seconds.

Add the coconut flour and coriander stalks and give it all a good stir. The pan will be looking a bit dry, so add the tomato purée and a little of the base sauce until you have a thick paste. Simmer for about 20 seconds, then add the remaining base sauce.

Allow this to come to a simmer, then stir in the coconut milk, chilli powder, mixed powder, tandoori masala and black pepper. Stir to combine and let it all bubble for about 3 minutes.

Add the tandoori chicken tikka or raw chicken and simmer in the sauce until heated through (or if using raw chicken, cooked through – after about 5 minutes).

To finish, add the dried fenugreek leaves (kasoori methi) by rubbing the leaves between your fingers. Stir in the mango chutney and squeeze in the lime juice. Sprinkle with the garam masala and season with salt to taste. Garnish with the chopped coriander and enjoy.

CHICKEN TIKKA BEEF KEEMA CHILLI GARLIC

SERVES 2

A big batch of keema is usually prepared and cooked ahead of service at curry houses as it saves time. This recipe calls for such a small amount of keema that it's safe to cook just as the method below. There is so much going on in this recipe with lots of different textures and flavours. They all go so well together, which is one reason I like this low-calorie Balti so much.

PREP TIME: 10 MINS, PLUS
PRE-COOKED INGREDIENT
TIME
COOKING TIME: 10 MINS

1 tbsp rapeseed (canola) oil
6 garlic cloves, thinly sliced
½ onion, finely chopped
1 tbsp garlic and ginger paste
2 green chillies, sliced into thin
　rings, plus extra to serve
　(optional)
½ tsp Kashmiri chilli powder
1 tbsp tandoori masala (see page
　148)
½ tbsp mixed powder (see page
　150) or curry powder
80g (2¾oz) lean beef mince or
　equivalent
70ml (¼ cup) tomato purée (see
　page 146)
300ml (1¼ cup) low-calorie base
　sauce (see page 82)
3 pieces of tandoori chicken
　tikka (see page 102)
A pinch of dried fenugreek
　leaves (kasoori methi)
Salt, to taste
1 tbsp finely chopped coriander
　(cilantro)

Heat the oil in a frying pan over a medium heat. Stir in the garlic and sizzle in the oil until a very light brown. Be careful not to burn it or it will taste bitter. Transfer to a plate.

Using the same oil, fry the onion for about 5 minutes until soft and translucent. Reduce the heat if the onion begins to burn. Stir in the garlic and ginger paste and green chillies and fry for 30 seconds, then add the ground spices and minced beef. Fry for about 1 minute or a little longer to brown the meat if using raw mince, then stir in the tomato purée, half the base sauce and the fried garlic. Bring to a simmer, only stirring if the sauce looks like it is sticking to the pan.

Add the chicken and the remaining base sauce and bring back to a simmer. When the chicken is heated through and the consistency of the sauce is to your liking, add the dried fenugreek leaves (kasoori methi) by rubbing the leaves between your fingers into the sauce. Season with salt and garnish with the coriander and a few more sliced chillies if you wish.

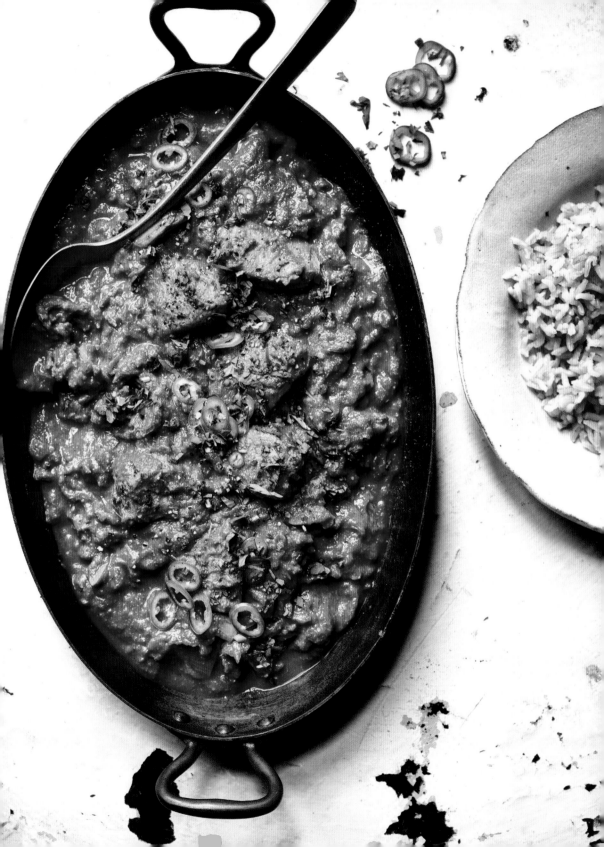

CHICKEN & BROCCOLI KORMA

SERVES 2

This popular mild curry is made much lighter here by using whisked yoghurt rather than cream and adding extra vegetables.

PREP TIME: 10 MINS, PLUS PRE-COOKED
INGREDIENT TIME
COOKING TIME: 10 MINS

1 tbsp rapeseed (canola) oil or melted ghee
½ cinnamon stick
Seeds from 2 green cardamom pods
½ tsp garlic and ginger paste
¾ tsp sugar or artificial sweetener (see page 8), to taste
5 cashew nuts, pounded to a paste with a little water
300ml (1¼ cups) low-calorie base sauce (see page 82)
150g (5½oz) raw chicken breast, cut into 5mm (¼-inch) slices
100g (3½oz) broccoli, cut into small florets
50g (1¾oz) block coconut, cut into small pieces
¾ tsp garam masala (see page 146)
50g (1¾oz) low-fat plain natural yoghurt, whisked until smooth and creamy
¼ tsp rosewater
Salt, to taste

Heat the oil in a large frying pan over a medium–high heat. When visibly hot, add the cinnamon and cardamom and give it all a good stir. Allow to infuse into the oil for about 20 seconds, then stir in the garlic and ginger paste. Sizzle until fragrant, about 20 seconds. Add the sugar or sweetener, cashew paste and half the base sauce. Let this come to a bubbling simmer, then stir in the chicken. Simmer for about 3 minutes until the chicken is almost cooked through, then add the broccoli.

Add the block coconut, garam masala and the remaining base sauce. Simmer for about 5 minutes until the chicken is cooked through and the broccoli is done to your liking.

Stir the yoghurt into the sauce, one tablespoon at a time. Add the rosewater and salt. If you prefer a sweeter sauce, add a little more sugar to taste.

CHICKEN CHASNI

SERVES 2

This curry is often quite sweet. I have reduced the amount of ketchup and chutney I would normally use to reduce the sugar content. If you find that it isn't sweet enough, add a little artificial sweetener to taste.

PREP TIME: 5 MINS, PLUS PRE-COOKED
INGREDIENT TIME
COOKING TIME: 10 MINS

1 tbsp rapeseed (canola) oil or light cooking spray
1 tsp garlic and ginger paste
¼ tsp ground turmeric
300ml (1¼ cups) low-calorie base sauce (see page 82), heated
200g (7oz) tandoori chicken tikka (see page 102)
2½ tsp smooth mango chutney
2½ tsp tomato ketchup
1½ tsp mint sauce
¾ tsp ground cumin
70g (2½oz) low-fat plain yoghurt
Juice of ½ lemon
Salt, to taste
About ½ tsp red food colouring powder (optional)

Heat the oil in a frying pan over a medium heat. Add the garlic and ginger paste and fry for about 25 seconds, to cook off the raw flavour. Add the turmeric and about a third of the base sauce. Bring to a simmer, then add the chicken. Stir it around in the sauce, then add the rest of the base sauce. Only stir if it looks like the sauce is sticking to the pan and scrape any that caramelizes on the side into the sauce. Stir in the mango chutney, ketchup, mint sauce and cumin and simmer for another minute, or until you are happy with the consistency. Whisk in the yoghurt one tablespoon at a time until the sauce is creamy-smooth.

Squeeze in the lemon juice and season with salt. This curry is usually bright red, which is done with food colouring powder. If that is the look you are going for, stir it in now. The colouring adds no flavour to the curry, so it is optional.

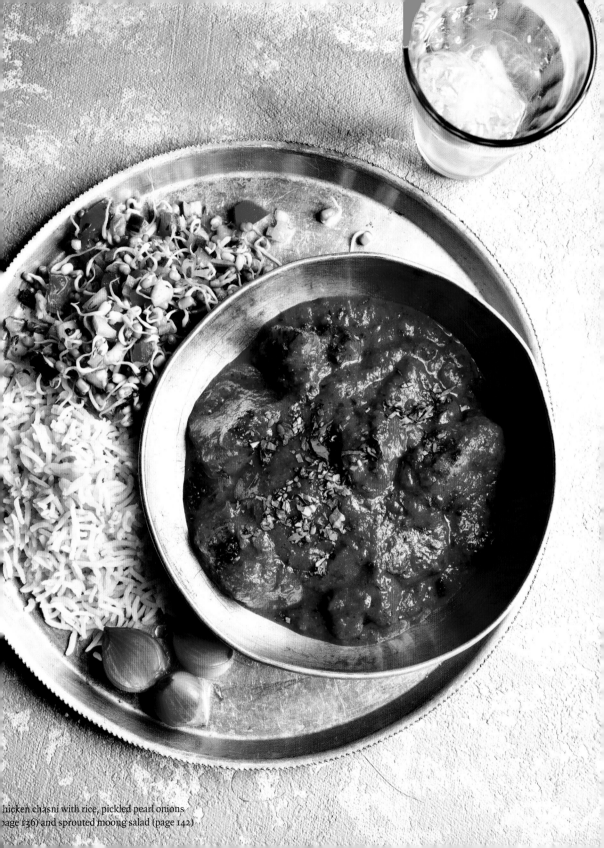

chicken chasni with rice, pickled pearl onions (page 136) and sprouted moong salad (page 142)

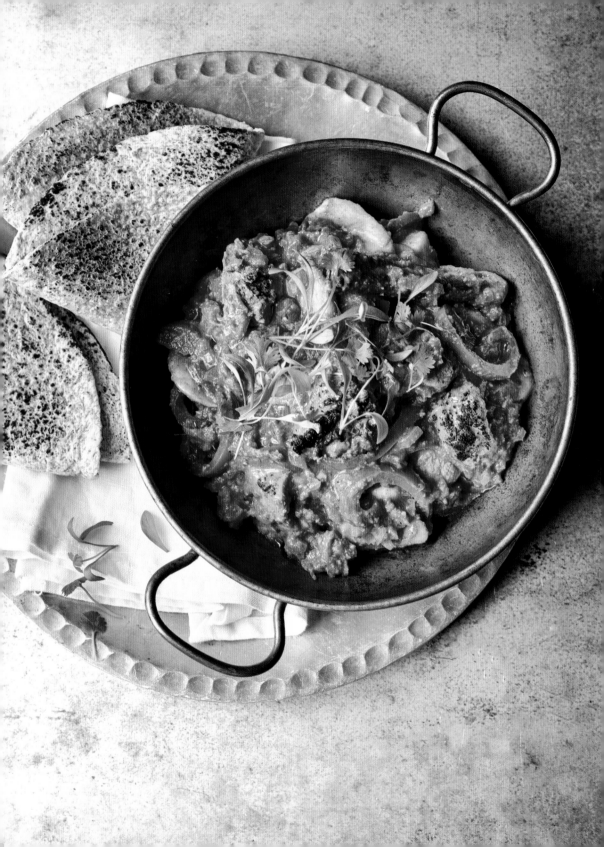

KASHMIRI CHICKEN (NO BASE SAUCE METHOD)
SERVES 2

Banana in a curry? I have to say that the first time I was offered a Kashmiri chicken curry, I wasn't convinced I would like it. As strange as it might sound to some, it was really good! I decided to make this recipe without a base sauce so that you could see how to make each of these curry-house curries without the prepared sauce. As you can see, it does take more time as the base sauce is a really convenient timesaver. If you would like to try this with the base sauce, just skip sautéing the onion and tomatoes and don't add the water. Use 300ml (1¼ cups) of low-calorie base sauce instead (see page 82), as with the other curry-house recipes. When you don't use a base sauce, you lose the curry-house flavour and texture, but the curry is still very nice.

PREP TIME: 10 MINS, PLUS
PRE-COOKED INGREDIENT
TIME
COOKING TIME: 20–25
MINS

1 tbsp melted ghee or rapeseed (canola) oil
½ cinnamon stick
Seeds from 3 green cardamom pods
2 cloves
1 onion, very finely chopped
1 tbsp garlic and ginger paste
2 medium tomatoes, diced
½ green (bell) pepper, sliced
1½ tsp mixed powder (see page 150) or curry powder
½ tsp Kashmiri chilli powder
200ml (¾ cup) water
1 tsp tamarind paste (see page 149) or concentrate
200g (7oz) tandoori chicken tikka (see page 102) or raw chicken breast, cut into bite-sized pieces
2 tbsp ground almonds
2 tsp smooth mango chutney
½ banana, sliced
3 tbsp low-fat plain yoghurt
Salt, to taste
Coriander (cilantro), to garnish

Heat the oil in a large frying pan over a medium heat. When hot, add the cinnamon stick, cardamom seeds and cloves and let them infuse into the oil for about 30 seconds. Add the onion and fry for about 6 minutes until soft and translucent. Stir in the garlic and ginger paste, tomatoes and green pepper and fry for another minute.

Now add the mixed powder and chilli powder and give it a good stir. Pour in the water and tamarind paste or concentrate and simmer over a medium–high heat for about 10 minutes until the onion and tomatoes break down into the sauce. Add the chicken, ground almonds and mango chutney and stir to coat the chicken. If needed, add a little more water. When the chicken is heated through (or if using raw chicken, cooked through – after about 5 minutes), stir in the banana and continue to simmer until you are happy with the consistency. To finish, whisk in the yoghurt, one tablespoon at a time. Season with salt and garnish with the coriander.

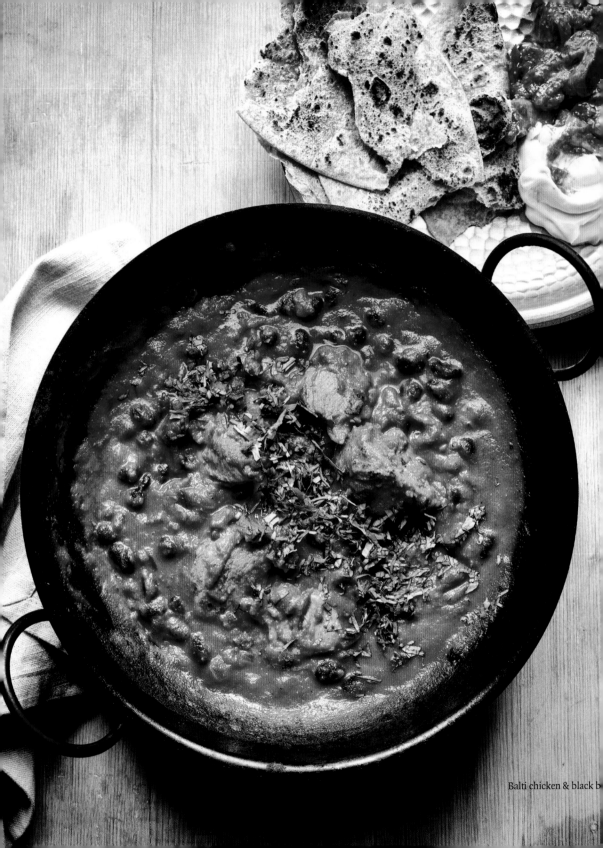

Balti chicken & black b

BALTI CHICKEN & BLACK BEANS
SERVES 2

Baltis are usually cooked over a very high heat with a lot of oil. The oil burns off quickly after it does its job, but here we'll stick to a small amount. If you have a Balti bowl, use it for this and serve it in the bowl it was cooked in.

PREP TIME: 5 MINS, PLUS PRE-COOKED
INGREDIENT TIME
COOKING TIME: 10 MINS

1 tbsp rapeseed (canola) oil
1/3 onion, finely chopped
1 1/2 tsp garlic and ginger paste
1/2 tsp ground cumin
1/2 tsp Kashmiri chilli powder
2 tsp mixed powder (see page 150) or curry powder
3 tbsp tomato purée (see page 146)
250ml (1 cup) low-calorie base curry sauce (see page 82)
100g (3 1/2oz) tandoori chicken tikka (see page 102) or
    raw chicken
400g (14oz) tinned (canned) black beans, drained
    (about 250g/9oz drained weight)
Salt, to taste
1 tbsp chopped coriander (cilantro), to garnish
Hot sauce or raita of your choice, to serve

Heat the oil in a frying pan over a medium–high heat. When bubbling hot, stir in the onion and fry for about 3 minutes until soft. Add the garlic and ginger paste and the ground spices, followed by the tomato purée. Bring to a simmer and pour in half the base sauce. Bring to a simmer, only stirring if the sauce is sticking to the pan. If any of the sauce caramelizes to the side, stir it in.

Add the chicken. If you are using tandoori chicken and have juices from the meat, stir them in for extra flavour. Stir in the remaining base sauce and the black beans and bring to a rolling simmer. When the meat is heated through (or if using raw chicken, cooked through – about 5 minutes), season with salt and garnish with the coriander. Serve with hot sauce or a good raita of your choice.

SAAG PANEER
SERVES 2

This veggie favourite is packed with healthy ingredients. The creamy spinach sauce with the soft, hot cheese is what does it for me.

PREP TIME: 5 MINS, PLUS PRE-COOKED
INGREDIENT TIME
COOKING TIME: 10 MINS

160g (5 3/4oz) baby spinach leaves
2 green chillies, roughly chopped
3 tbsp roughly chopped coriander (cilantro)
70ml (1/4 cup) water
1 tbsp rapeseed (canola) oil
1 tsp cumin seeds
1/4 cinnamon stick
1/2 onion, finely chopped
A pinch of salt
2 tsp garlic and ginger paste
1 tsp mixed powder (see page 150) or curry powder
70ml (1/4 cup) tomato purée (see page 146)
200ml (3/4 cup) low-calorie base curry sauce (see page 82)
70g (2 1/2oz) paneer, cubed
Juice of 1 lemon, or to taste
A pinch of dried fenugreek leaves (kasoori methi)
Salt, to taste
1/2 tsp garam masala (see page 146)

Blend the spinach, chillies, coriander and water into a smooth paste. Set aside.

Heat the oil in a frying pan over a medium heat. When hot, add the cumin and cinnamon and fry for about 30 seconds to infuse the flavours. Add the onion and salt and fry for about 4 minutes until soft and translucent. Stir in the garlic and ginger paste and fry for a further 30 seconds, then add the mixed powder, tomato purée and half the base sauce. Simmer, stirring only if the sauce is sticking. If any sauce caramelizes to the side, stir into the sauce for extra flavour. As it thickens, stir in the remaining sauce and the spinach mixture. Return to a simmer, then stir in the paneer.

Simmer until the paneer is heated through and you are happy with the consistency. Squeeze in the lemon juice and dust with the dried fenugreek leaves (kasoori methi). Season with salt and the garam masala. Serve hot.

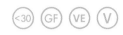

302KCAL

34.7G CARBS

VEGETARIAN KEBABI MADRAS

SERVES 2

Kebabis are simply small pieces of seekh kebab. Here I use the corn and potato kebabs, which work really well and make a tasty vegetarian madras. As with all the curry-house-style curries in this book, feel free to add or substitute as you please. Meat fans will love this with the meat kebab (see page 111) cut into small bite-sized pieces. If you happen to have some good stock to hand, add a few tablespoons of that for extra flavour.

PREP TIME: 5 MINS
COOKING TIME: 10 MINS

1 tbsp rapeseed (canola) oil
1 dried Kashmiri chilli
2 green cardamom pods, smashed
1 tbsp garlic and ginger paste
1 green bird's eye chilli, cut into thing rings (more or less, to taste)
150ml (¾ cup) tomato purée (see page 146)
¾ tbsp ground cumin
1 tsp ground coriander
1 tbsp mixed powder (see page 150) or curry powder
¾ tbsp Kashmiri chilli powder (more or less, to taste)
300ml (1¼ cups) low-calorie base curry sauce (see page 82)
1 tsp smooth mango chutney or lime pickle
200g (7oz) grilled corn and potato kebab, cut into bite-sized pieces (see page 111)
Juice of ½ lemon
Salt, to taste
2 tbsp finely chopped coriander (cilantro), to garnish
A pinch of garam masala (see page 146)

Heat the oil in a frying pan over a medium–high heat. Add the dried chilli and cardamoms and let them infuse into the oil for about 30 seconds. Stir in the garlic and ginger paste and green chilli and fry for a further 20 seconds, then add the tomato purée. Stir well, then add the ground spices. As this comes to a bubble, stir in about half the base curry sauce and bring to a rolling simmer. Only stir if the sauce is obviously sticking to the pan. If it begins to caramelize to the sides of the pan, stir this into the sauce.

Add the mango chutney and the rest of the base sauce. Bring to a simmer, then add the vegetable kebabis. Just heat them through – do not overcook them or they will fall apart in the sauce. To serve, squeeze in the lemon juice and season with salt. Garnish with the coriander and a pinch of garam masala.

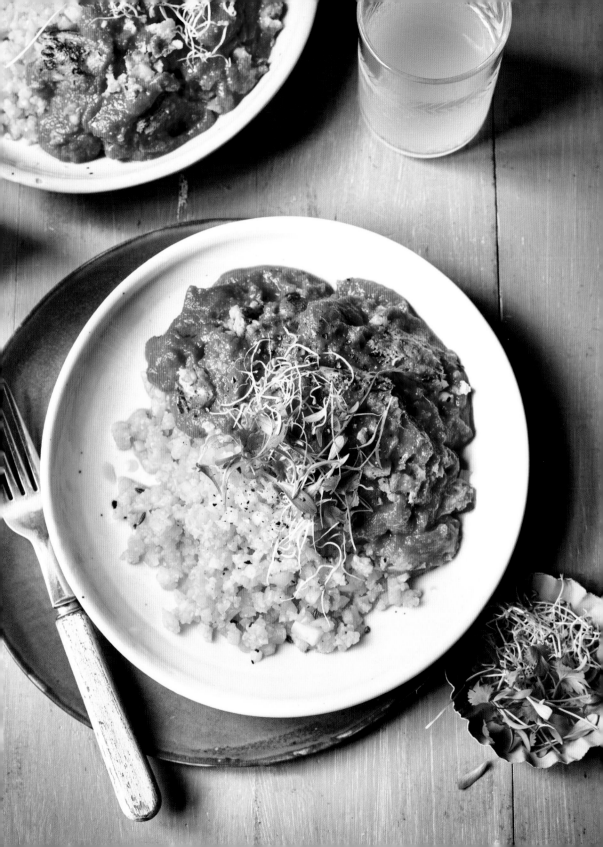

LIGHT & DELICIOUS BARBECUE

Barbecuing and grilling are perfect for cooking light meals.
Cooking over hot coals means you need to use far less oil,
and there's nothing wrong with that. This chapter gives you
all the information you need to ensure these easy barbecue
recipes go right for you. The information on the page
opposite will help get you started.

PREPARING YOUR BARBECUE FOR DIRECT HEAT COOKING

Cooking over open flames is the simplest of the three methods used in this section. When your food is exposed to the intense direct heat, it gets a wonderful, smoky char on the exterior, while the interior remains deliciously juicy.

When preparing your charcoal, it is a good idea to build a two-level fire. Tip the charcoal into the basin of the barbecue, then spread the charcoal so that two-thirds of the coals are stacked about twice as high as the remaining one-third. This way, you can easily move whatever it is you're cooking from the hot side of the grill to the cooler side if it begins to burn before it's cooked through.

I use a lot of charcoal: about two full shoe boxes. It is important to achieve that intense heat. Light the charcoal and let it heat up until the coals are white-hot. To check if the coals are ready, hold your hand about 5cm (2 inches) above the grill or cooking level if using skewers; if your hand becomes uncomfortably hot in two seconds, you're ready start grilling.

I like to cook using flat skewers. Skewering meat, seafood, paneer and vegetables gives the finished dish that authentic tandoori restaurant look. You could also use a grill.

PREPARING YOUR BARBECUE FOR INDIRECT HEAT COOKING

This method is used for roasting, and you will need a barbecue that has a tight-fitting lid. Fill the barbecue on one side only with about two shoe boxes full of charcoal, leaving the other half empty. Light a few fire starters and pile in the charcoal. Let it heat until white-hot. Place the grill on top and whatever it is you're cooking over the side with no coals. Cover and cook. If you are barbecuing for a long period of time, you will need to throw a few handfuls of charcoal on the fire every 30 minutes or so.

OVEN COOKING

Ovens vary, but I usually crank mine up to 200°C (400°F/Gas 6) and cook the meat on a wire rack near the top. To get that charred appearance and flavour, place the roasted meat at the end of cooking under a hot grill for a couple of minutes before serving.

LIGHT TANDOORI CHICKEN TIKKA
SERVES 6

You don't need a lot of fat to make tandoori chicken taste amazing. What, with all those spices? This chicken is delicious served simply on its own, but I have to recommend making it to use in your curries. That's one of the things that makes British Indian restaurant-style food so good. You could cook this chicken in the oven, but I prefer the smoky flavour of the barbecue. Whichever you decided, this one you have to make. It goes well with the sliced red onion salad on page 141.

PREP TIME: 10 MINS, PLUS
MARINATING TIME
COOKING TIME: 10 MINS

1kg (2lb 4oz) skinless, boneless
    chicken breasts, cut into bite-
    sized pieces
Juice of 2 lemons
3 tbsp garlic and ginger paste
1 tsp flaky sea salt
Red food colouring powder
    (optional)

FOR THE MARINADE
250g (1¼ cups) fat-free Greek
    yoghurt
1 tbsp ground cumin
1 tbsp ground coriander
2 tbsp tandoori masala (see page
    148)
1 tsp amchoor (dried mango
    powder)
1 tsp ground turmeric
1 tsp Kashmiri chilli powder
1 tbsp green chilli paste or
    2 green chillies, finely
    chopped
20g (¾oz) coriander (cilantro),
    finely chopped
Salt, to taste

Place the chicken in a large mixing bowl and drizzle the lemon juice over the top. Mix in the garlic and ginger paste, salt and red food colouring (if using). Allow to stand while you make the marinade.

Place the yoghurt in a large mixing bowl and whisk in the remaining ingredients except the salt until creamy smooth. Add the chicken pieces and rub the marinade into the flesh. The chicken needs to marinate for at least 30 minutes, but a few hours or overnight will get you tastier results.

When ready to cook, set up your barbecue for direct heat cooking (see page 101). Skewer the chicken pieces onto five or six skewers. If you are using the tandoori chicken in a creamy curry, such as chicken tikka masala, be sure to retain the marinade. Whisking in 1–2 tablespoons adds delicious flavour. When the coals are white-hot, place the skewers over the heat and grill for about 5 minutes until you get a good char on the underside. Flip over the skewers and cook the other side until nicely charred and cooked through. Season with salt and serve.

If you would rather cook your tandoori chicken tikka in the oven, preheat it to 200°C (400°F/Gas 6). Place the chicken tikka on a rack in the middle of the oven and cook for about 20 minutes, turning once, halfway through cooking. The chicken is ready when the juices run clear when pricked with a fork. You can also get that grilled, charred look by placing the cooked chicken under a hot grill for a couple of minutes.

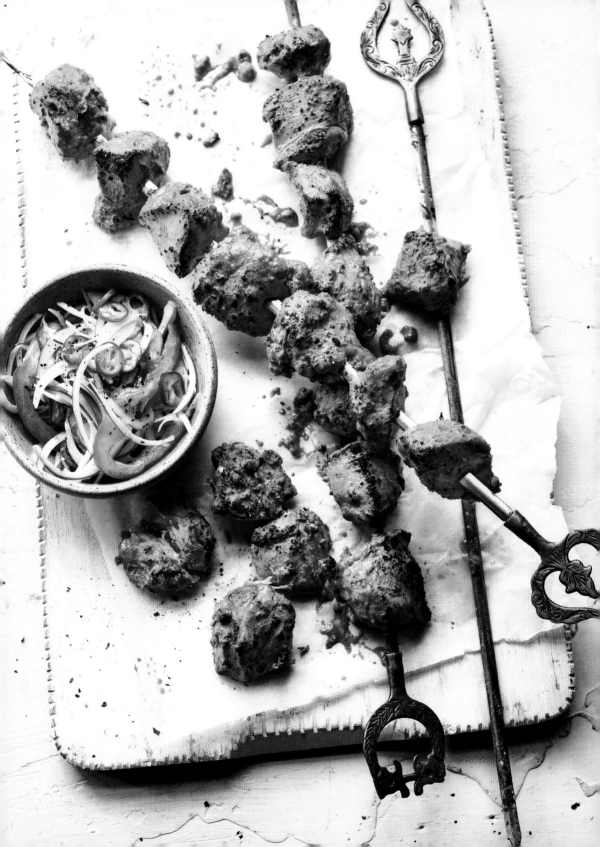

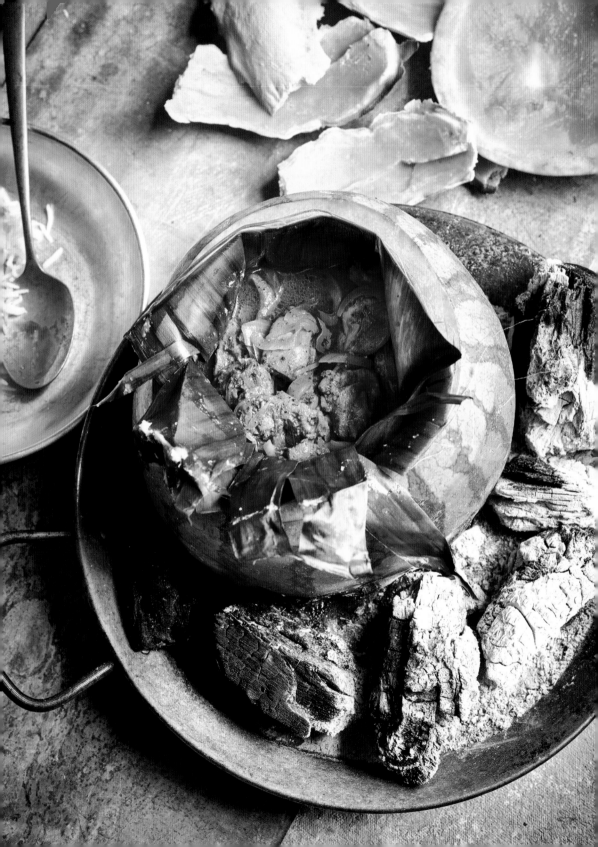

WATERMELON COCONUT CHICKEN CURRY
SERVES 4

This recipe was inspired by Indian tribal cooking, where the watermelon is used as a cooking vessel, but I think the flavour is better if you cook it on the hob before heating it up in the melon. I first tried curry prepared in this way when my wife and I stayed at Lake Canopy Resort in Kerala. Their talented head chef at the time, Vipin VU, sent this out to our table, and I just had to get the recipe for you! This is great served with plain basmati or matta rice (see page 123).

PREP TIME: 20 MINS, PLUS
MARINATING TIME
COOKING TIME: 40 MINS

500g (1lb 2oz) chicken breasts or
  thighs, skinned and cut into
  bite-sized pieces

FOR THE MARINADE
1 tbsp lemon juice
½ tsp Kashmiri chilli powder
¼ tsp ground turmeric
½ tsp garam masala (see page 146)
½ tsp freshly ground black
  pepper

FOR THE SPICE PASTE
1½ tbsp coriander seeds
½ cinnamon stick
4 cloves
Seeds from 2 green cardamom
  pods
8 black peppercorns
¾ tsp fennel seeds
¼ tsp cumin seeds
½ tsp Kashmiri chilli powder

FOR THE SAUCE
2 tbsp rapeseed (canola) oil
10 fresh or frozen curry leaves
2 medium onions, thinly sliced
1 tbsp garlic and ginger paste
250ml (1 cup) light coconut milk
Salt, to taste

FOR THE WATERMELON
1 medium watermelon
250g (2 cups) plain (all-purpose)
  flour
225ml (scant 1 cup) water
1 large banana leaf (optional)

Place the chicken in a bowl with the marinade ingredients and stir well to combine. Set aside for at least 30 minutes.

For the special spice paste, dry-fry the whole spices in a frying pan, stirring them around in the pan so that they toast evenly until they are fragrant and warm to the touch but not yet smoking. Transfer to a plate to cool, then blend with the Kashmiri chilli powder and just enough water – about 35ml (⅛ cup) – to make a smooth paste. Set aside.

To make the sauce, heat the oil in a large saucepan over a medium–high heat and stir in the curry leaves and onions and fry for about 5 minutes until the onions are soft and translucent. Stir in the garlic and ginger paste and fry for a further 30 seconds. Now add the marinated chicken and fry for about 3 minutes until it turns white in colour. Add the spice paste and stir it all up to combine. Add the coconut milk and bring to a simmer, then cover and simmer for a further 5 minutes. Season with salt. The curry is ready if you're not heating it on the barbecue in the melon.

Set up your barbecue for indirect heat cooking (see page 101). Cut off the top of the watermelon and hollow it out, placing the melon chunks in the fridge (the cooled watermelon pieces make a nice light dessert). Mix the flour and water together to make a workable dough. You won't be eating this; it is used only to seal the seam between the bottom of the watermelon lid, which you cut off to empty it. If using the banana leaf, which adds flavour, wash it well, then line the inside of the watermelon with it. Tip the curry into the melon and place the lid back on top. Roll out the dough into a long rope and press it against the seam to seal it. Make a well in the coals so that it looks like a big charcoal doughnut. Stand the watermelon in a heatproof serving bowl and place it right down in the coals. Cover the barbecue and cook for about 15 minutes until the dough is blackened on the outside.

To serve, place a few burning coals around the watermelon and place at the table. Carefully slice away the dough at the top and lift the lid.

GRILLED CHICKEN CAFREAL
SERVES 4

The original cafreal is believed to have been brought to Goa by the Portuguese. The Portuguese first learned to make it in their African colonies, and the Goans learned to make it from them and the African sailors who worked on their ships. As with so many Goan recipes, I'm sure they made a few changes to the original to make it their own. Many say that it is a green version of piri piri, which also originated in Africa. The marinated chicken is usually fried, but I like to char it on the barbecue and then simmer the par-cooked chicken in the marinade over hot coals. Although this is a very famous chicken dish, the marinade goes equally well with fish, vegetables and paneer. This curry is delicious served with brown rice and/or a simple mixed green salad. In Goa, it is often served with deep-fried and battered potato slices; I recommend serving it with my much healthier cumin potatoes on page 126.

PREP TIME: 15 MINS, PLUS MARINATING TIME
COOKING TIME: 20 MINS

1 generous tbsp black peppercorns
8 cloves
½ cinnamon stick, broken into small pieces
1 tsp cumin seeds
1 tsp coriander seeds
1½ tsp ground turmeric
100g (3½oz) very fresh coriander (cilantro) leaves and stalks, roughly chopped
5 green chillies, roughly chopped (more or less, to taste)
10 garlic cloves
5cm (2-inch) piece of ginger, peeled and roughly chopped
Juice of 1–2 limes
1.2kg (2lb 10oz) chicken, skinned and cut into eight pieces, or 700g (1lb 9oz) boneless chicken thighs
1 tsp rapeseed (canola) oil or cooking spray
70ml (¼ cup) coconut vinegar or malt vinegar
Salt, to taste
2 long red chillies, cut into rings, to garnish
3 tbsp finely chopped coriander (cilantro), to garnish

Heat a dry frying pan over a medium heat and toast the whole spices until fragrant and warm to the touch, but not smoking. Transfer the spices to a bowl to cool, then grind them to a fine powder in a spice grinder or pestle and mortar and stir in the ground turmeric. Place the fresh coriander, chillies, garlic, ginger and lime juice in the spice grinder or pestle and mortar and pound or grind to a thick green paste. If you need a little more liquid to help with the blending, add some of the vinegar.

Cut a few shallow slits in each piece of chicken using a sharp knife. Place the chicken in a large glass bowl and rub the coriander paste into it, ensuring it is well coated. Cover and refrigerate for at least 30 minutes or overnight – the longer the better.

When ready to cook, set up your barbecue for direct heat cooking (see page 101). Brush the grill with the rapeseed oil or spray it with cooking spray. When really hot, remove as much of the marinade from the chicken as possible, but do not discard the marinade. Grill the chicken pieces on one side for about 3 minutes, or until it begins to char, then flip over to char the other side.

When the chicken is nicely charred but not completely cooked through, place a saucepan or wok on the grill. Put the charred chicken pieces in the pan. Clean the bowl that the chicken was marinating in with about 125ml (½ cup) of water, mixing all the leftover marinade into the water. Add the vinegar, then pour this liquid over the chicken in the pan. Simmer for 5–10 minutes until the chicken is completely cooked through and you have a nice thick, green sauce.

To serve, place the chicken on a plate and spoon the cooking sauce over it. Season with salt and garnish with the chillies and coriander.

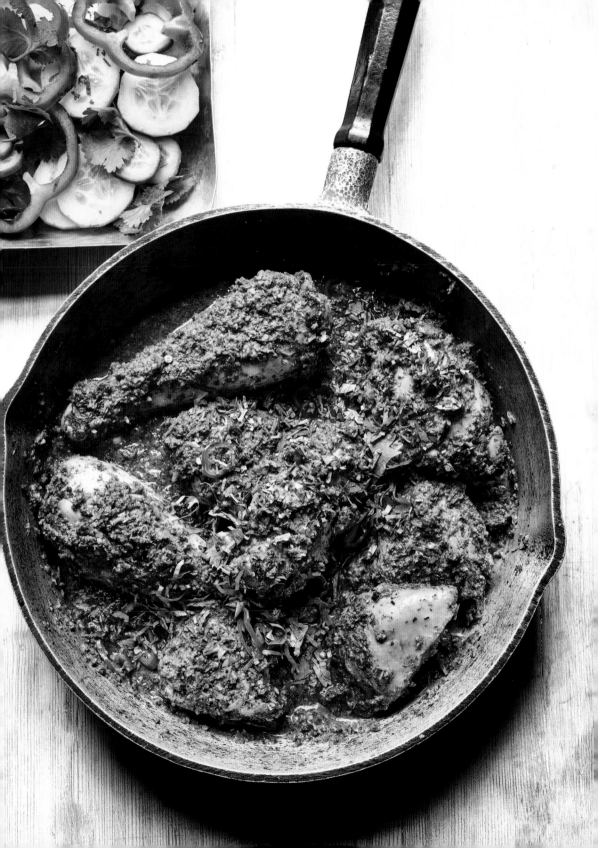

EASY TANDOORI CHICKEN THIGHS

SERVES 4

I think you're going to like this simple marinade. It is another way that tandoori chicken is prepared at some takeaways, and I really like it. Most of the ghee/vinegar mopping sauce drips into the coals, giving the chicken its characteristic smoky flavour. On the topic of flavour, thigh meat has a lot more of it than chicken breasts. It's cheaper and tastes better and is my cut of choice when barbecuing chicken. You can serve this with a light green salad, or if you plan a few days ahead, you could also enjoy it with the sprouted moong salad on page 142.

PREP TIME: 15 MINS, PLUS
MARINATING TIME
COOKING TIME: 10 MINS

8 chicken thighs on the bone,
   skinned
3 tbsp white malt vinegar
¾ tbsp Kashmiri chilli powder
1 tbsp rapeseed (canola) oil, plus
   a little extra for grilling
2 tbsp garlic and ginger paste
1 tsp salt

FOR THE YOGHURT
MARINADE

300g (1½ cups) fat-free Greek
   yoghurt
2 red chillies, pounded to a paste
   in a pestle and mortar or
   finely chopped
2 tbsp tandoori masala (see page
   148) or garam masala (see
   page 146)
Salt, to taste

FOR BASTING

3 tbsp white malt vinegar
2 tbsp melted ghee
1 tbsp tandoori masala or garam
   masala

Make three shallow slits in each chicken thigh and place them in a large mixing bowl. Add the vinegar, Kashmiri chilli powder, oil, garlic and ginger paste, and salt and mix well with your hands. Set aside while you make the yoghurt marinade.

In a separate bowl, whisk the yoghurt until creamy smooth, then add the remaining marinade ingredients. Pour over the chicken and mix it all evenly over the chicken thighs. Leave to marinate for at least 30 minutes or overnight – the longer the better.

When ready to cook, mix all the basting ingredients together in a small bowl and keep it handy. Brush the grill with oil or spray it with a little cooking spray. Set up your barbecue for direct heat cooking (see page 101). When the coals are white-hot, place your hand about 5cm (2 inches) over the grill. If your hand is unbearably hot after two seconds, you're ready to start cooking.

Remove as much of the marinade as possible from the chicken and place the thighs on the grill. Cook for 5 minutes until browned on the underside, then flip over. Grill for another 5 minutes, basting from time to time with the basting liquid – you don't need to use it all up! Check for doneness and flip over again if necessary. The chicken is ready when pierced with a fork or sharp knife and the juice runs clear. If you have a meat thermometer, chicken should be cooked to 75°C (167°F).

TANDOORI LAMB CHOPS
SERVES 4

The marinade for these lamb chops is a great all-round marinade that is good for making tandoori meat tikka with cubed lamb, mutton or beef. This recipe makes enough to marinate up to 800g (1lb 12oz) meat tikka, which is delicious served with a salad, wrapped into a chapatti and/or cooked into a curry house-style curry (see pages 80–99.) Here it's used for lamb chops, which are so good on the barbecue. They also aren't as calorific as you might think!

PREP TIME: 20 MINS, PLUS
MARINATING TIME
COOKING TIME: 10 MINS

8 lamb chops, all excess fat
   trimmed off
Rapeseed (canola oil) or cooking
   spray, for brushing
1 tbsp melted ghee, for basting
(optional)

FOR THE FIRST MARINADE
2 tbsp lemon juice
2 tbsp garlic and ginger paste
½ tsp Kashmiri chilli powder
½ tsp salt

FOR THE SECOND
MARINADE
2 tbsp garlic and ginger paste
½ tsp chilli powder
½ tsp ground turmeric
½ tsp salt
1 tsp garam masala (see page
   146) or tandoori masala (see
   page 148)
1 tsp ground cumin
1 tsp ground coriander
2 tbsp lemon juice
3 generous tbsp fat-free Greek
   yoghurt

Whisk all the ingredients together for the first marinade in a large bowl and add the lamb chops. Make sure they are completely coated in the marinade and set aside for 20 minutes.

Whisk all the ingredients for the second marinade in a separate bowl and add the marinated lamb chops. Leave for at least 30 minutes or overnight – the longer the better.

When ready to cook, set up your barbecue for direct heat cooking (see page 101). Spray the grill with cooking spray or brush it with a little oil. When the coals are white-hot and your hand is unbearably hot after placing it 5cm (2 inches) above the grill for two seconds, you're ready to cook.

Place the lamb chops on the grill and cook for 5 minutes, then flip them over. Cook for a further 3–5 minutes, or until cooked to your liking. If you like, you can lightly baste the chops with ghee during cooking for an additional 16 calories per chop. I think it's worth the calories, but you might not.

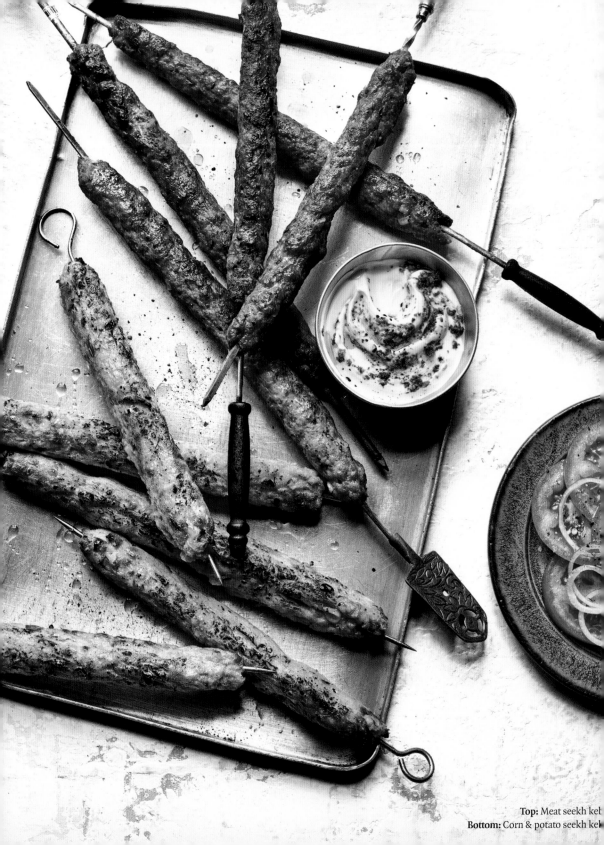

Top: Meat seekh keb
Bottom: Corn & potato seekh keb

MEAT SEEKH KEBABS

SERVES 4

This uses lean mince rather than the fatty meat you get at many takeaways.

PREP TIME: 15 MINS
COOKING TIME: 8 MINS

1 egg
800g (1lb 12oz) lean lamb mince or other lean mince
1 tbsp garlic and ginger paste
1 tbsp ground coriander
1 tsp Kashmiri chilli powder
1 tsp freshly ground black pepper
½ tsp ground turmeric
1 tbsp garam masala (see page 146) or tandoori masala (see page 148)
½ onion, finely chopped or grated
1 tsp salt
3 tbsp finely chopped coriander (cilantro) or mint
Cooking spray, or rapeseed (canola) oil, for brushing

Whisk the egg in a large bowl, then add the remaining ingredients except the cooking spray or oil. Mix well with your hands, then place on a clean work surface or large plate. Knead the meat for about 5 minutes, pushing it down and across the surface with the palms of your hands. You should see streaks of meat being left behind on the surface.

Set up your barbecue for direct heat cooking (see page 101). If cooking on the grill, brush it with a little oil or spray it with cooking spray. When the coals are white-hot and your hand is unbearably hot after placing it 5cm (2 inches) above the grill for two seconds, you're ready to cook.

Grease the skewers lightly with oil. Take a piece of mince no larger than a pool ball and push it onto the skewer. Forming the meat into a sausage shape, working the meat down the skewer until it is even in width and secure.

Place over the fire or on the grill and cook until lightly browned on one side, then flip over and lightly brown the other side. As there is little fat, you don't want to overcook them. Serve hot when the meat is cooked to your liking.

CORN & POTATO SEEKH KEBABS

SERVES 4

The kebabs are delicious served on their own with a little chutney or used in a curry, as in the vegetable kebabi madras on page 98.

PREP TIME: 10 MINS
COOKING TIME: 40 MINS

3 corn on the cob or 200g (7oz) tinned (canned)
175g (6oz) mashed potato
2 spring onions (scallions), finely chopped
2 green bird's eye chillies, finely chopped
1 tbsp gram flour
1 tsp garam masala (see page 146)
Salt, to taste
Cooking spray, for greasing
1 tbsp melted ghee (optional)
½ tsp Kashmiri chilli powder or chaat masala (see page 148)

If using tinned (canned) corn, finely chop it. It is already cooked, so it's ready to use. If using corn on the cob, boil in water for about 20 minutes, then drain. Allow the cobs to cool a little, then grate the corn off the cobs. To make the mashed potato, boil 175g (6 oz) of potatoes until they are fall-apart tender, then mash.

Place the corn and mashed potato in a mixing bowl and add the rest of the ingredients up to and including the garam masala. Season with salt.

Divide the corn mixture into four balls. Lightly oil the skewers with cooking spray, then firmly form the kebabs onto the skewers. Squeeze them on with your hand so that there is no movement.

When ready to cook, set up your barbecue for direct heat cooking (see page 101). When the coals are good and hot, place the skewers over the fire and cook, turning from time to time until toasty brown all over. This should only take about 5 minutes. Season with salt and lightly brush with the ghee (if using). Sprinkle with the Kashmiri chilli powder or chaat masala to serve.

GRILLED TUNA STEAKS WITH WATERMELON & PINEAPPLE SALSA
SERVES 4

This is such an easy dish to prepare and I love the combination of flavours. I sometimes make a simple butternut squash purée to go with this dish. Try blending the butternut squash curry on page 72 and you won't be disappointed. This recipe was inspired by a recipe shown to me by my friend Chef Shihabudeen VM. It's a winner!

PREP TIME: 10 MINS, PLUS
MARINATING TIME
COOKING TIME: 5 MINS

4 x 200g (7oz) thickly cut tuna
    steaks
½ tsp salt
1 tsp freshly ground black
    pepper
1 tsp Kashmiri chilli powder
½ tsp ground turmeric
1 generous tsp garlic and ginger
    paste
1 tbsp white malt vinegar
1 tbsp rapeseed (canola) oil
Salt, to taste
A few slices of red onion, to
    garnish
1 lime, sliced, to garnish

FOR THE SALSA
100g (3½oz) watermelon, diced
100g (3½oz) pineapple, diced
2 green chillies, finely sliced
3 spring onions (scallions),
    thinly sliced
1 tbsp green olives, roughly
    chopped
1 tbsp black olives, roughly
    chopped
Salt, to taste

Take the tuna steaks out of the fridge 30 minutes before cooking. Mix the salt, black pepper, Kashmiri chilli powder, ground turmeric, garlic and ginger paste, vinegar and oil in a mixing bowl. Place the tuna steaks in the bowl and be sure to coat them all over with the marinade. Set aside.

To make the salsa, mix the watermelon, pineapple, chillies, spring onions and green and black olives together in a mixing bowl. Season with salt to taste.

Set up your barbecue for direct heat grilling (see page 101). When the coals are white hot and it is uncomfortably hot for you to hold your hand 5cm (2 inches) above the grill, you are ready to cook. Place the tuna steaks on the grill and cook for 2 minutes and then flip over to cook for a further 2 minutes. This should produce a nice char while being nice and pink in the middle. Transfer to heated plates when you are happy with the doneness.

To serve, season each steak with salt to taste and then top with the watermelon and pineapple salsa. Garnish with red onion and lime.

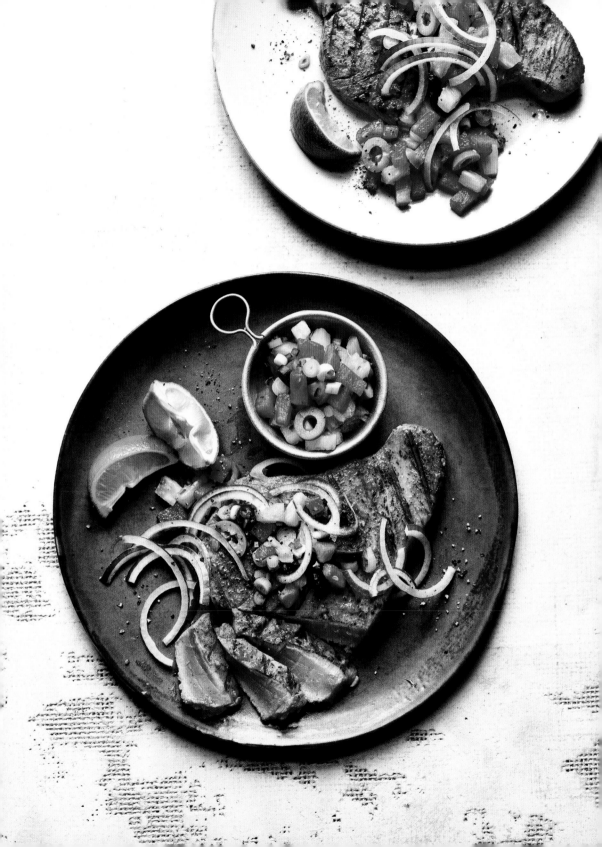

BAMBOO COOKED SEAFOOD

SERVES 2

This is a fun way of barbecuing a curry, and it's a really healthy way of cooking too. You could go out and purchase bamboo shoot steamers or save yourself a lot of money and just purchase a couple of large, untreated bamboo fence posts online or at larger DIY shops. Then cut them up into short segments to use like this. Of course, you could make this curry by wrapping it up in foil or a banana leaf, but place the package further away from the fire. The thick bamboo doesn't only add flavour but also protects the curry from burning in the heat. This curry is great served with matta rice (see page 123) and a green salad, like the moong sprout salad on page 142.

PREP TIME: 15 MINS, PLUS
SOAKING TIME
COOKING TIME: 8 MINS

2 x roughly 20cm (8-inch)
   bamboo shoots, about 10cm
   (4 inches) in diameter
2 tbsp melted coconut oil
1 tsp ground turmeric
2 tbsp garlic and ginger paste
3 green chillies, finely chopped
10 fresh or frozen curry leaves,
   finely chopped
2 tbsp lime juice
½ tsp salt, plus more to taste
1 tsp freshly ground black
   pepper
2 shallots, thinly sliced
500g (1lb 2oz) mixed seafood
   like cod, squid, halibut,
   salmon, etc.
6 tbsp fresh or frozen grated
   coconut
240g (2 cups) plain (all-purpose)
   flour
250ml (1 cup) water

Submerge and soak the bamboo shoots in water for about 1 hour. When ready to cook, set up your barbecue for direct heat cooking (see page 101). In a mixing bowl, combine two teaspoons of the melted coconut oil with the rest of the ingredients up to and including the coconut and mix well. Set aside for about 10 minutes.

In a separate bowl, mix together the flour and water until you have a soft dough. You won't be eating this – it will hold the seafood in the bamboo as it cooks. Use the remaining coconut oil to lightly grease the inside of the bamboo, then use the dough to seal one end of a bamboo pole and fill with half the seafood mixture. Seal the other end with more dough. Repeat with the other pole.

Place the bamboo cookers right down in the coals. On page 4 you will find a photograph of this being done. Cook for 8 minutes, then remove from the coals using tongs. Be careful as they will be hot! Tip the contents over hot rice or into warmed plates.

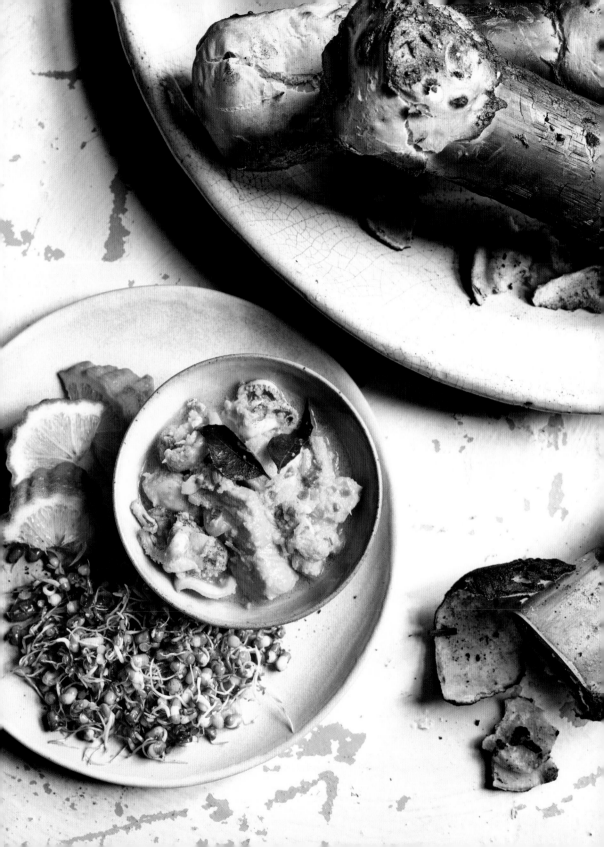

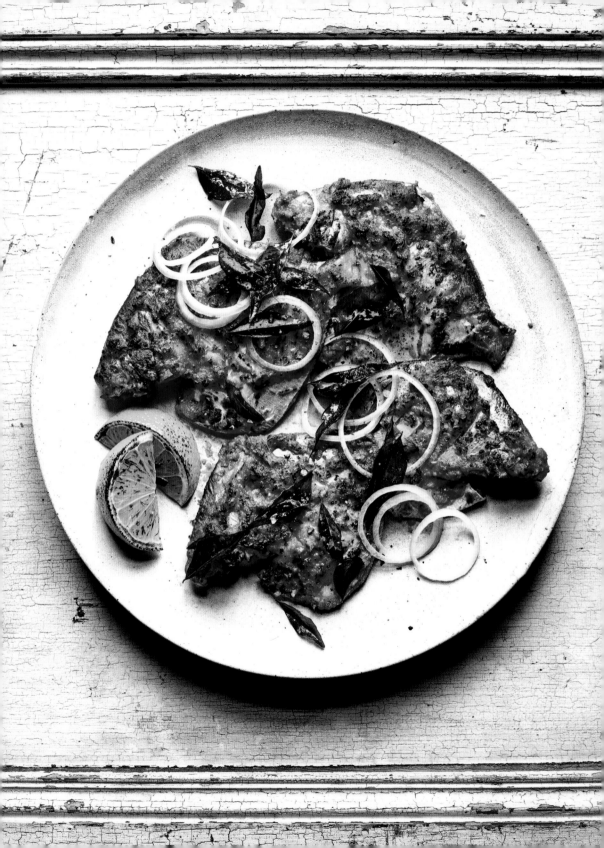

CHEF JOMON'S TANDOORI POMFRET
SERVES 4

This recipe is a bit of a mix of north and south Indian cooking. My good friend, Jomon Kuriakose, Chef de Cuisine at the Lalit in London, was born and raised in Kerala, where he learned to cook and shop for ingredients from his mother. One of his favourite dishes was her pan-fried pomfret using special blends of Keralan spices. One day, his fishmonger here in the UK sent him some silver pomfret to try and it brought back memories of his favourite dish. Having also been influenced here in the UK by tandoor cooking, which is more of a northern Indian style of cooking, he decided to try his mum's recipe – not fried but cooked in the tandoor with mustard oil. The result, which you can try for yourself, is amazing! No worries if you don't have a tandoor, it's also delicious cooked on the barbecue! Frozen pomfret are available at many Asian shops and also from online fishmongers. There's no substitute, but this recipe does work really well with lemon sole and sea bass too.

PREP TIME: 10 MINS, PLUS MARINATING TIME
COOKING TIME: 15 MINS

4 silver pomfret (gutted and cleaned)
2 tsp Kashmiri chilli powder
½ tsp ground turmeric
1 tsp crushed black pepper
30 fresh or frozen curry leaves
1 mango, peeled, pitted and roughly chopped
3 shallots
6 garlic cloves
2.5cm (1-inch) piece of ginger, peeled and minced
2 tbsp mustard oil
1 tsp rapeseed (canola) oil
1 lemon, cut into wedges
Flaky sea salt, to taste
Red onion slices, to garnish

Place the cleaned pomfret on a cutting board and score each side three to five times. Using a spice grinder or blender, blend the Kashmiri chilli powder, turmeric, black pepper, 20 of the curry leaves, the mango, shallots, garlic, ginger and the mustard oil to a smooth paste. Gently rub the paste inside and outside the fish and leave to marinate for 2–3 hours.

To make the curry-leaf garnish, heat the rapeseed (canola) oil in a frying pan and, when hot, lightly fry the remaining curry leaves until shiny and a bit crispy. Set aside for later.

When ready to cook, set up your barbecue for indirect heat cooking (see page 101). Place the fish on the grill and cook for 10–15 minutes, or until the fish is cooked through. Alternatively, you could set up your barbecue for direct heat cooking (see page 101), skewer the fish onto metal skewers and cook right over the coals, turning once for a more charred finish.

To oven cook, preheat the oven to 200°C (400°F/Gas 6) and place the marinated fish on a baking tray. Cook for 10–15 minutes on the top rack, turning the fish once. Baste once or twice during cooking.

If you like, you could char the lemon wedges for the garnish, or you could just serve them fresh.

To finish, season the fish with salt to taste and place one fish on each of four heated plates. Garnish with the curry leaves, onion slices and lemon wedges.

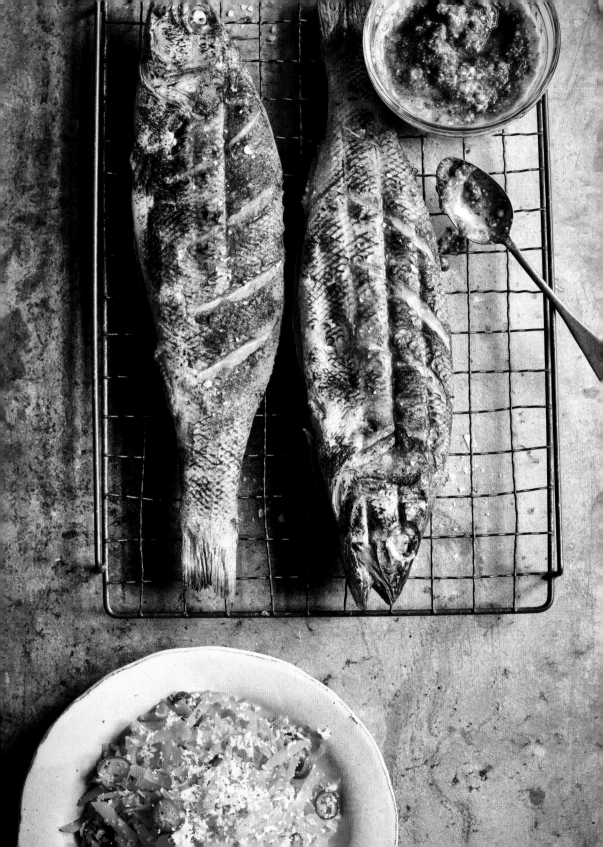

GRILLED SEA BASS WITH GREEN CHILLI & CORIANDER SAUCE

SERVES 4

I used to pan-fry the sea bass for this recipe and still do from time to time. I do like the flavour of the charred skin you get from grilling over hot coals and hey... barbecuing is fat-free cooking! The low-calorie green sauce is served on the side and it's so nice to dip the grilled fish in it – or drown it in the sauce – depending on your mood and flavour preference. Although not essential, a barbecue fish holder will come in very handy for this recipe. I like to serve this dish with my carrot and coconut salad on page 142.

PREP TIME: 15 MINS
COOKING TIME: 40 MINS

FOR THE SAUCE
1 large onion, roughly chopped
15 cashew nuts
500ml (2 cups) water
2.5cm (1-inch) piece of ginger,
    peeled and roughly chopped
5 garlic cloves, smashed
3 green bird's eye chillies,
    roughly chopped (more or
    less, to taste)
50g (1¾oz) coriander (cilantro)
1 tbsp rapeseed (canola) oil
1 tsp ground turmeric
Juice of 1 large lemon
Salt and freshly ground black
    pepper, to taste

FOR THE FISH
4 medium 250g (9oz) whole sea
    bass, cleaned and scored every
    1.5cm (½-inch)
1 tsp ground turmeric
Salt and freshly ground black
    pepper, to taste
Cooking spray or rapeseed
    (canola) oil
2 lemons, quartered

Start by making the sauce. Put the onion and cashew nuts in a saucepan with 250ml (1 cup) of the water and simmer over a medium heat for about 20 minutes. Blend to a paste, then transfer to a bowl.

Meanwhile, blend the ginger, garlic, chillies and coriander with just enough water (about 70ml/¼ cup) to make a thick paste. Set aside.

Heat the oil over a low heat and add the onion and cashew paste and cook, stirring regularly, for 10 minutes. Pour in the remaining water along with the turmeric, lemon juice and blended coriander paste. You can either pass it all through a fine-mesh sieve or leave it as is. Season with salt and black pepper, then pour the sauce into four dipping bowls.

To cook the sea bass, set up your barbecue for direct heat cooking (see page 101). Rub the turmeric all over the fish and season with salt and black pepper. When ready to cook, place the fish in a fish holder sprayed with cooking spray or lightly greased with oil and place it over the fire. Cook for about 3 minutes per side, or until the fish is cooked through. Serve with lemon wedges and the green sauce.

SPICY STUFFED CRABS

SERVES 4

One of my favourite meals when I visit Goa is masala-stuffed crab. There, they use small blue crabs or freshwater mud crabs, but we can't get these where I live. So for this recipe, I use dressed brown crabs. Ordering dressed crabs from your fishmonger takes away most of the work needed to make this recipe. In the warmer months, I usually purchase my crabs live, then boil and clean them and pick out all the meat before proceeding with this recipe and cooking them on the barbecue. Brown crab has a lot of wet, brown meat that needs to be thickened. Shop-bought dressed crabs are often thickened with bread crumbs, but if using live crabs, you could cook them and then thicken them with cooked grated potato. Substitute polenta for the semolina and you have a gluten-free version of this recipe. Obviously, if eating light isn't something that concerns you, you could always add more oil and butter. Personally, I don't think you'll miss the fat with this recipe. There are so many delicious spices and other ingredients in the mix.

PREP TIME: 10 MINS
COOKING TIME: 30 MINS

1 tbsp rapeseed (canola) oil
1 large onion, finely chopped
3 green chillies, finely chopped
10 fresh or frozen curry leaves, roughly chopped
4 garlic cloves, minced
½ tsp ground turmeric
1 tsp chilli powder
3 tbsp cider vinegar or coconut vinegar
3 tbsp finely chopped coriander (cilantro)
Salt, to taste
4 dressed brown crabs
1 egg, beaten with 1 tbsp water
3 tbsp coarse semolina
1 tbsp melted butter

Heat the oil in a large non-stick frying pan over a low–medium heat. Fry the onion for 8–10 minutes, stirring often, until soft and translucent. As we are using a small amount of oil, you will need to watch the onion carefully so that it doesn't burn. Stir in the green chillies, curry leaves, garlic and the ground spices and stir to combine. Fry for a further 30 seconds and stir in the vinegar and coriander. Season with salt. This is a good time to adjust spicing too, so add more chilli powder if you want to and/or more vinegar.

Remove the masala from the heat and pour it into a large bowl to cool. Add the crabmeat from the shells and stir well.

Set up your barbecue for indirect cooking (see page 101).

Transfer this masala crabmeat in equal amounts back into the crab shells. Lightly brush each crab with the egg wash – you won't use anywhere near as much as you have. Sprinkle each equally with the semolina and drizzle the butter over the top.

Place the crabs directly on the grill on the side without the coals. Cover and cook for 15–20 minutes or until heated through and lightly browned on top. Serve immediately.

NOTE

This can also be cooked in an oven. Preheat your oven to 200°C (400°F/Gas 6) and cook on a baking tray in the middle of the oven for 15–20 minutes until heated through.

LIGHT
SIDE DISHES

In this section you are sure to find what you are looking
for. These are sides that are healthy and for the most part
easy to make too. Rice is a main staple in south Indian
cooking, so I included a couple of my favourite recipes.
If you are on a low-carb or no-carb diet, I have also
included some excellent alternatives to rice.

You will also find my recipe for masala rotis, which
are amazing served on their own or loaded with
vegetables, meat or paneer.

This selection of stir-fried vegetables, raitas, pickles and
chutneys offers a mouth-watering way to liven up a meal.

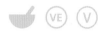
MASALA ROTI
MAKES 10

Leave all the spices out and you have plain chapattis. Go ahead and have a play with this one, adding the spices you want; cumin and coriander are always nice. Try to keep the spices you use to a minimum or the flavour will be a bit too complicated. The key to making perfect rotis is to get them evenly rolled out and as round as possible. This takes practice, but your first attempts will still be amazing!

PREP TIME: 10 MINS, PLUS
SITTING TIME
COOKING TIME: 15 MINS

200g (1½ cups) chapatti flour,
  plus extra for dusting
1 tsp salt
¼ tsp ground turmeric
½ tsp Kashmiri chilli powder
1 tsp garam masala (see page
  146)
½ tsp freshly ground black
  pepper
190ml (generous ¾ cup) hot
  water

Tip the flour, salt and the ground spices into a mixing bowl and stir to combine. Make a small well in the middle with your hand, then slowly start pouring in the water. Work the mixture until you have a soft dough, transfer to a clean work surface, then knead into a ball. The dough should be slightly sticky to the touch and easy to knead. If too sticky, add a bit more flour. Knead the dough for at least 5 minutes, then transfer to the bowl and cover with a damp cloth for at least 30 minutes.

When ready to cook the rotis, divide the dough into 10 equal-sized balls. Take a ball and flatten it with your hand onto a lightly floured surface. Roll it out, working the rolling pin in a clockwise direction and paying attention to make the roti as round and evenly flat as you can. The end roti should be thin like you would expect a chapatti to be. Repeat with the remaining dough balls.

Heat a frying pan over a medium–high heat. Take the first roti and dust off any excess flour as this will burn. Place it in the pan and as the underside cooks, bubbles will appear on top. This should take 30–45 seconds. When this happens, flip the roti over to cook the other side for about 30 seconds. Flip it over again and press the areas between the small bubbles with a damp tea (dish) towel or spatula. This will help make bubbles larger and if you're lucky it will puff right up like a balloon. If you have a gas hob, place the roti right on the fire to finish, which will also help it puff up and become lighter. Repeat with the remaining rotis and keep warm.

NOTE

Making perfect rotis takes practice. If you cook on too low a temperature, the roti will become crisp; if too high, it will burn in some places and remain raw in others. The roti should puff up like a balloon, but if it doesn't, it will still be good. Just get it to bubble up as best you can for lighter rotis.

363KCAL
51.8G CARBS

GOAN COCONUT RICE

SERVES 6

I'm a big fan of coconut rice, and this is one of the easiest recipes I know. Although it takes over an hour to make, there isn't much work to do. This is an excellent way to get the flavour of Goan coconut rice without even breaking open one coconut! It is perfect with any of the curry recipes in this book.

PREP TIME: 30 MINS, PLUS SOAKING TIME
COOKING TIME: 45 MINS

370g (13oz) basmati rice
2 tbsp coconut oil
1 cinnamon stick
3 cardamom pods, smashed
2 cloves
2 x 400ml (14fl oz) cans light coconut milk
Salt, to taste

Place the rice in a mixing bowl and cover with water. Using your hand, swirl the rice around in the water until it becomes milky in colour. This is the starch that you need to get rid of before cooking. Carefully pour the water out and refill. Repeat this process several times until the water runs almost clear. Leave the rice to soak for 30 minutes, then drain completely.

Melt the coconut oil in a large saucepan that has a tight-fitting lid. Add the whole spices and temper them in the oil over a medium heat for about 30 seconds. Tip in the rice and coat it well in the seasoned oil. Pour in the coconut milk, cover and bring to a boil over a high heat. When the coconut milk boils, turn off the heat and leave for 40 minutes. Do not be tempted to lift the lid.

After 40 minutes, lift the lid and gently stir the rice with a fork to separate the grains. If you do this too vigorously, the rice will turn to mush, so be careful. Season with salt and serve immediately.

 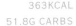

229KCAL
47.3G CARBS

AROMATIC MATTA RICE

SERVES 6

I know white basmati rice tastes amazing, but matta rice is much healthier for you and equally delicious. I first tried it in Goa where it is called Goan red rice, but most matta rice is grown in Kerala, where it's called, you guessed it... Keralan red rice. The red colour of the rice is the outer pericarp, which is removed from processed white rice, leaving it with little nutritional value. I have to say I now prefer matta rice to plain white rice because of its earthy flavour and the fact that it is full of vitamins and fibre. It also leaves you feeling fuller while eating less!

PREP TIME: 5 MINS, PLUS SOAKING TIME
COOKING TIME: 30 MINS

370g (13oz) matta rice (available online and from Asian grocers)
1.5 litres (6¼ cups) water
½ tsp salt
1 cinnamon stick
5 black peppercorns
5 cloves

Rinse the rice in a large bowl in several changes of water until the water runs clear. Soak the rinsed rice for 30 minutes–1 hour. When ready, bring the water with the salt and spices to a boil in a large saucepan. Drain the rice, add it to the pan and cook for about 20 minutes, or until tender. Some brands take longer to cook, so read the packet instructions. The rice is ready when you can squish a grain of rice between your fingers, but it should not be at all mushy. When in doubt, try it. The rice should be enjoyable to eat and still have a bit of a bite to it.

Drain the rice through a sieve and leave to drain for about 5 minutes. Serve with any curry or dhal of your choice.

BROCCOLI RICE

SERVES 4

Both broccoli and cauliflower rice offer an excellent way to get those veggies in and make equally satisfying substitutes for rice. This simple recipe could be used with cauliflower too. Vegetable 'rice' like this can be eaten on its own but also offers a delicious, low-calorie way to soak up a good curry. If you'd like to jazz it up a bit, try the cauliflower rice pilau, using cauliflower and/or broccoli.

PREP TIME: 10 MINS
COOKING TIME: 4 MINS

1 large head of broccoli, cut into florets
1 tbsp rapeseed (canola) oil or melted coconut oil
Salt and freshly ground black pepper, to taste

Using a cheese grater or food processor, grate or blend the broccoli until it looks like rice. Place the broccoli rice in a microwave-safe bowl, stir in the oil and cover lightly with plastic wrap. Microwave for 2 minutes, then give it a good stir. Cover again and cook for a further 1–2 minutes until tender. Season with salt and black pepper.

CAULIFLOWER RICE PILAU

SERVES 4

This is a pimped-up version of broccoli rice. You can use broccoli and/or cauliflower.

PREP TIME: 10 MINS
COOKING TIME: 15 MINS

1 medium–large head of cauliflower or 450g (1lb) store-bought cauliflower rice
2 tbsp rapeseed (canola) oil
55g (½ cup) sliced almonds
1 cinnamon stick
2 green cardamom pods, smashed
3 garlic cloves, minced
Pinch of dried red chilli flakes
1 small bunch of coriander (cilantro), finely chopped
1 tbsp lemon juice
Salt and freshly ground black pepper, to taste

If working with a head of cauliflower, cut it into small pieces. You can remove the core if you wish. Place it in a food processor and pulse until the cauliflower chunks look like rice.

Cauliflower contains a lot of water so wrap the cauliflower rice in a thin, clean tea (dish) towel and twist it into a ball. As you wrap it tightly, it will begin to release excess water. This will give the cauliflower a nicer and drier appearance when cooked.

Heat 1 teaspoon of the oil in a large frying pan over a medium–high heat and fry the almonds for about 3 minutes until lightly browned. Take care not to burn them. Transfer to a bowl and set aside.

In the same pan, heat the remaining oil over a medium–high heat, then add the cinnamon and cardamom pods and let them infuse in the oil for about 30 seconds. Add the garlic and fry for about 30 seconds more. Add the cauliflower rice and dried red chilli flakes and stir well to combine. Continue frying, stirring regularly, until the cauliflower is hot and turns a light golden brown in places. This should take about 7 minutes.

To finish, stir in the almonds, coriander and lemon juice. Season with salt and black pepper.

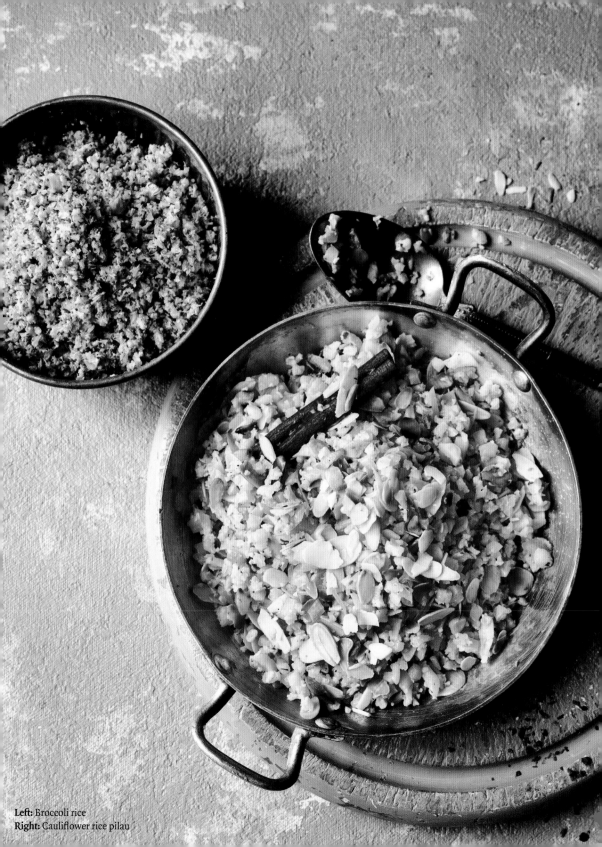

Left: Broccoli rice
Right: Cauliflower rice pilau

(<30) (VE) (V)

(GF) (VE) (V)

CUMIN POTATOES
SERVES 2

RED LENTIL & TOMATO DHAL
SERVES UP TO 8

Talk about easy! I cook this one all the time, even if I'm not cooking an Indian meal. Cumin potatoes are an excellent substitute for the more fatty Sunday lunch roast potatoes. You might have seen these at Indian restaurants (called jeera aloo). Whatever you call them, they make the perfect side for so many dishes; I like to serve them with a good raita to dip the potatoes into and perhaps a small chapatti.

PREP TIME: 5 MINS
COOKING TIME: 20 MINS

3–4 medium potatoes (about 300g/11oz), skin on
½ tbsp rapeseed (canola) oil or ghee
1½ tsp cumin seeds
2 green chillies, finely chopped
Salt, to taste
2 tbsp chopped coriander (cilantro), to garnish
Juice of ½ lemon

Bring a saucepan of water to the boil and cook the potatoes for about 15 minutes, or until soft and completely cooked through. Allow to cool slightly, then peel and chop them into small bite-sized pieces.

Heat the oil in a frying pan over a medium–high heat and add the cumin seeds. When they begin to crackle, reduce the heat to low and add the green chillies and fry for about 45 seconds. Add the potatoes and stir well to combine. Season with salt.

To serve, garnish with the coriander and drizzle the lemon juice over the top.

One good thing about this Goan recipe dhal is that it cooks really quickly – a lot faster than other dhals – and still tastes fantastic. This makes a lovely side dish but can also be a delicious and light main meal on its own.

PREP TIME: 10 MINS, PLUS SOAKING TIME
COOKING TIME: 25 MINS

2 tbsp rapeseed (canola) oil or coconut oil
1 tsp black mustard seeds
½ tsp cumin seeds
7 fresh or frozen curry leaves
2 medium onions, finely chopped
2 medium tomatoes, diced
2–3 green bird's eye chillies, sliced down the middle
2 tbsp garlic and ginger paste
1 tsp ground turmeric
1 tsp Kashmiri chilli powder (more or less, to taste)
3 tbsp tomato purée (see page 146)
300g (1½ cups) dried red split lentils (masoor dhal), rinsed and soaked for 30 minutes in fresh water
1.2 litres (5 cups) water
Salt, to taste
2 tbsp finely chopped coriander (cilantro)

Heat the oil in a large saucepan over a high heat. When visibly hot, stir in the mustard seeds. When they begin to pop (after about 30 seconds), reduce the temperature to medium–high and add the cumin seeds and curry leaves. Temper for 30 seconds, or until fragrant, then add the onions and fry for about 5 minutes, until soft and translucent.

Add the tomatoes, green chillies, garlic and ginger paste, ground turmeric, Kashmiri chilli powder and tomato purée and give it all a good stir to combine. Tip in the lentils and cover with the water. Bring to a simmer and cook for 15–20 minutes, or until the lentils are soft and you are happy with the consistency.

Season with salt and garnish with the coriander to serve.

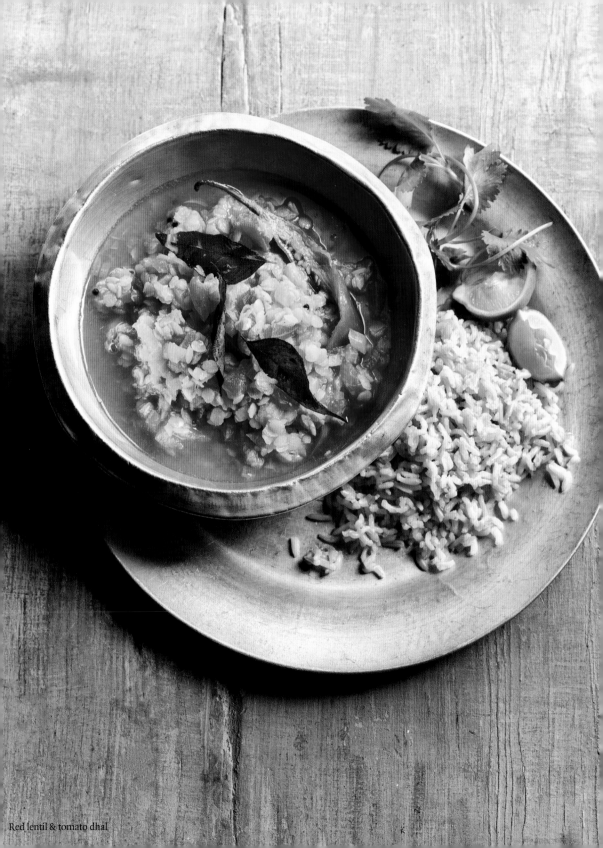

Red lentil & tomato dhal

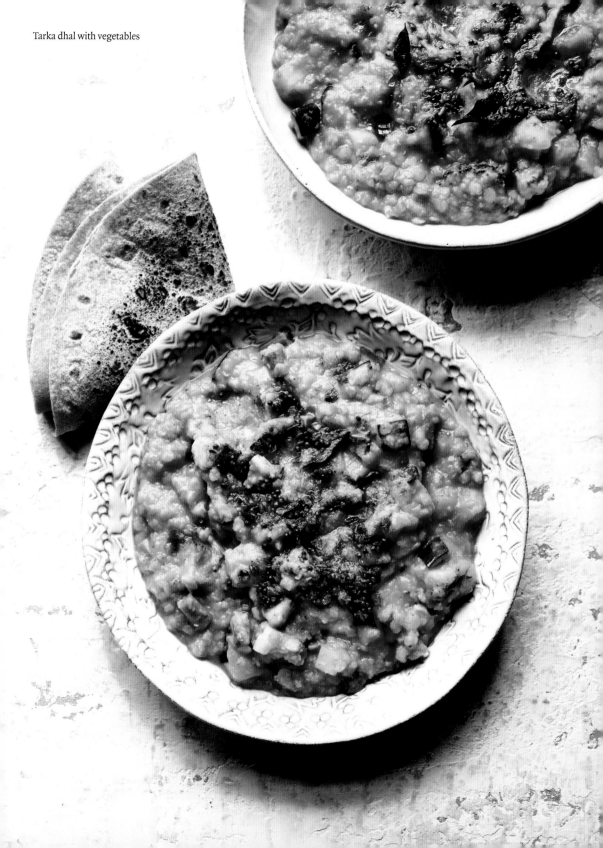

Tarka dhal with vegetables

TARKA DHAL WITH VEGETABLES
SERVES 8

This recipe is great as a side or delicious simply served over white rice as a main meal.

PREP TIME: 10 MINS
COOKING TIME: 25 MINS

250g (1½ cups) massoor dhal, rinsed and soaked in water for 30 minutes
50g (1¾oz) each of roughly chopped carrot, potato cut into small cubes, broccoli florets, green beans cut small, aubergine cut small, or whatever sounds good
2 tbsp ghee or rapeseed (canola) oil
½ tsp black mustard seeds
1 tsp cumin seeds
½ cinnamon stick
10 fresh or frozen curry leaves
1 tbsp garlic and ginger paste
1 tbsp garam masala (see page 146)
¼ tsp Kashmiri chilli powder (optional)
½ tsp ground turmeric
Salt and freshly ground pepper, to taste

Tip the lentils into a saucepan and pour in about 400ml (scant 1¾ cups) of water. Simmer over a medium heat for about 10 minutes and skim off any foam that rises to the top. Add the carrot and potato pieces and continue cooking for another 5 minutes before adding the rest of the veggies. Stir the vegetables in, adding more water only if the lentils are looking dry, and cook until the vegetables are cooked through and the lentils are fall-apart soft. Keep warm.

Meanwhile, heat the ghee in a small frying pan over a medium–high heat. When it bubbles, add the black mustard seeds and when they begin to crackle (after about 30 seconds), reduce the heat to medium and stir in the cumin seeds, cinnamon stick and curry leaves. Fry for about 30 seconds, then add the garlic and ginger paste, garam masala, Kashmiri chilli powder (if using) and turmeric. Fry for another 30 seconds, then pour it over the cooked lentils. Season with salt and black pepper and serve.

GREEN BEAN FUGATH
SERVES 4

This is a quick one to make and an excellent vegetable side dish to serve with any curry or barbecued dishes. I love the combination of the green beans and coconut. I like to cook the beans until just cooked through so that they still have a good bite to them.

PREP TIME: 5 MINS
COOKING TIME: 10 MINS

1 tbsp coconut oil or rapeseed (canola) oil
½ tsp black mustard seeds
10 fresh or frozen curry leaves
1 medium red onion, halved, finely sliced and cut into 2.5cm (1-inch) pieces
2 green chillies, sliced lengthways
300g (11oz) green beans, cut into 1cm (¾-inch) pieces
½ tsp ground turmeric
50g (1¾oz) fresh or frozen grated coconut
Salt, to taste

Heat the oil in a large frying pan over a high heat. When visibly hot, add the black mustard seeds. When they begin to pop (after about 30 seconds), stir in the curry leaves and fry for about 30 seconds until fragrant. Add the onion and chillies and fry for 2 minutes until the onion is just becoming soft, then add the green beans.

Stir well to combine, then add the turmeric and coconut. Pour in about 70ml (¼ cup) of water to help the green beans cook. When almost all the water has evaporated and the beans are cooked through, season with salt and serve.

130KCAL
8G CARBS

152KCAL
11.5G CARBS

CABBAGE FUGATH

SERVES 4

Cabbage fugath is a delicious side dish that I often serve with the bean fugath on page 129. Not only do they complement each other well, but many of the ingredients are the same, so you can prepare them together to save time.

PREP TIME: 5 MINS
COOKING TIME: 25 MINS

1 tbsp coconut oil or rapeseed (canola) oil
1 tsp black mustard seeds
10 fresh or frozen curry leaves
50g (1¾oz) fresh or frozen grated coconut
1 medium red onion, halved, finely sliced and cut into 2.5cm (1-inch) pieces
2 green chillies, sliced lengthways
2.5cm (1-inch) piece of ginger, peeled and finely chopped
450g (1lb) shredded green cabbage
Salt, to taste

Heat the oil in a large frying pan over a high heat. When visibly hot, add the black mustard seeds. When they begin to pop (after about 30 seconds), stir in the curry leaves and temper them in the oil for about 30 seconds. Add the coconut and fry, stirring regularly, for about 5 minutes until light brown. Add the onion and chillies and stir well. Reduce the heat to medium and fry the onion and chillies for about 5 minutes, or until the onion is soft and translucent. Stir in the ginger and cook for another minute.

Now it's time to add the cabbage. The pan will look very full, but the cabbage will reduce as it releases water. Stir it all up well to combine and then cover with a lid. Cook over a low heat for about 10 minutes until just soft but not soggy. Season with salt and serve.

STIR-FRIED BRUSSELS SPROUTS

SERVES 2

This dish uses water and oil for lighter sautéing. Oil makes cooking easier, and you could use more, but give this a try. You need to watch it closely, but will end up with crispy Brussels sprouts that taste fantastic.

PREP TIME: 10 MINS
COOKING TIME: 15 MINS

20 Brussels sprouts
1½ tsp rapeseed (canola) oil or coconut oil
1 tsp black mustard seeds
1 tsp cumin seeds
1 medium onion, finely chopped
1 green chilli, finely chopped
1 tsp finely chopped fresh ginger
2 garlic cloves, finely sliced
3 tbsp fresh or frozen grated coconut
Salt, to taste

Using a sharp knife, quarter the Brussels sprouts. Heat the oil in a frying pan over a medium–high heat. When the oil is visibly hot, add the black mustard seeds. When they begin to pop (after about 30 seconds), reduce the heat to medium and stir in the cumin seeds. Fry for a further 20 seconds or so until fragrant.

Add 2 teaspoons of water to the pan, then add the onion. Stir it all up well and sauté the onion until soft and glossy. You might need to add another teaspoon or so of water, but don't add too much or you will boil the onion instead of sautéing it.

When the onion is soft, after about 5 minutes, add the green chilli and ginger, along with the Brussels sprouts. Stir well to coat the sprouts in the onion mixture and sauté for about 5 minutes until the sprouts are cooked through. Only add a drop more water if the onion or sprouts are sticking to the pan. As the sprouts cook, they will crisp up. Add the garlic and coconut and sauté for 2 minutes until soft. Season with salt and serve.

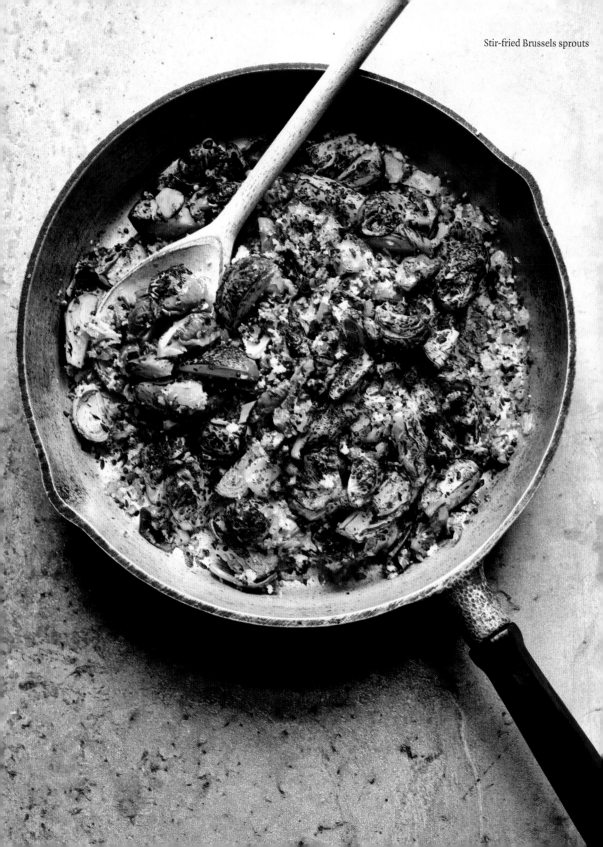

Stir-fried Brussels sprouts

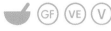

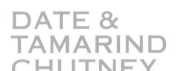

123KCAL PER TBSP
15.9G CARBS PER TBSP

MANGO, CHILLI & COCONUT SALAD

SERVES 4
PREP TIME: 10 MINS

3 mangos, peeled, pitted and sliced into cubes
Juice of 2 limes
1 tsp Kashmiri chilli powder (or to taste)
Flaky sea salt, to taste
3 tbsp finely chopped coriander (cilantro)
50g (1¾oz) shaved fresh coconut

Place equal amounts of mango on four plates. Squeeze the lime juice over the top and sprinkle with the Kashmiri chilli powder and salt.

Garnish with the coriander and coconut.

9KCAL PER TBSP
0.4G CARBS PER TBSP

CORIANDER & MINT CHUTNEY

MAKES ABOUT 250ML (1 CUP)
PREP TIME: 10 MINS

50g (1¾oz) coriander (cilantro) leaves
20g (¾oz) mint leaves
2 green chillies, roughly chopped
1 garlic clove, roughly chopped
1.5cm (½ inch) piece of ginger, peeled, finely chopped
5 cashew nuts
½ tsp chaat masala (see page 148)
½ tsp ground cumin
½ tsp ground coriander
Juice of ½ lime
Salt, to taste

Put all the ingredients up to and including the ground coriander in a blender. Add a drop of water and blend into a thick green paste. Stir in the lime juice and season with salt.

21KCAL PER TBSP
4.7G CARBS PER TBSP

DATE & TAMARIND CHUTNEY

MAKES ABOUT 600ML (2½ CUPS)

This is delicious and keeps for weeks in the fridge. It is quite high in natural sugars, so use sparingly. It is pictured on page 135.

PREP TIME: 10 MINS, PLUS SOAKING TIME
COOKING TIME: 1 HOUR

300g (11oz) soft, pitted dried dates
200g (7oz) block of tamarind
1¼ tsp salt
1 tsp black salt
½ tsp ground cumin
½ tsp ground coriander
1 tsp ground ginger
½ tsp Kashmiri chilli powder
Sugar or artificial sweetener, to taste (optional)

Soak the dates in water for 30 minutes, then drain.

Bring 300ml (1¼ cups) of water to the boil in a saucepan and break the tamarind into it. Simmer for about 10 minutes, then allow to cool. Squeeze the tamarind pulp in the water to break it up more, then run it through a fine-mesh sieve into a bowl, pushing the solids through and discarding the seeds and any larger pieces. You now have a paste that can be used whenever tamarind paste (or concentrate) is called for in a recipe.

Place the tamarind liquid in a blender with the soaked dates and blend into a fine paste. If you need to add a little water, that is fine.

Pour the tamarind and date liquid back into the saucepan, add another 500ml (2 cups) water and simmer on a low heat for about 45 minutes, until the sauce is just a little thinner than ketchup.

Stir in the salt, black salt, cumin, coriander, ginger and Kashmiri chilli powder. Simmer for a further 3 minutes to combine the flavours. Taste it – if you prefer a sweeter flavour, add a little sugar or sweetener to taste.

Transfer the hot chutney to a sterilized jar with a tight-fitting lid. Allow to cool completely, then screw on the lid and refrigerate.

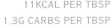
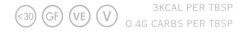
ROASTED TOMATO CHUTNEY

MAKES ABOUT 250ML (1 CUP)

Roasted tomato chutney is amazing used as a dip for crudités or papadams. It also makes a great marinade and sauce for grilled meats and fish. Try it with my recipe on page 119.

PREP TIME: 10 MINS
COOKING TIME: 15 MINS

5 medium–large tomatoes
50g (1¾oz) Bengal gram (chana lentils)
1 tsp rapeseed (canola) oil
1 tsp cumin
2 garlic cloves, smashed and roughly chopped
2 green chillies
3 tbsp chopped coriander (cilantro) leaves
1 tsp Kashmiri chilli powder
1 tsp chaat masala (see page 148)
½ tsp amchoor (dried mango powder)
2 generous tbsp low-fat Greek yoghurt
1 tsp lemon juice
Salt, to taste

Grill the tomatoes under the oven grill or, better still, directly over a gas or open fire flame until blackened. Turn them often so that they roast evenly. This should take about 5 minutes. Set aside to cool slightly, then dice them.

In a dry frying pan over a medium heat, toast the Bengal gram for about 5 minutes, stirring regularly until toasted and brown in colour. Transfer to a plate to cool.

Now add the oil to the pan and stir in the cumin and garlic and sauté for about 1 minute. Add the green chillies, coriander, Bengal gram and tomatoes and bring to a simmer. Add the Kashmiri chilli powder, chaat masala and amchoor (dried mango powder). Stir well and remove from the heat to cool slightly. Whisk in the yoghurt and blend to a smooth paste. Stir in the lemon juice and season with salt. Taste the chutney: if you find that it is too spicy, stir in more yoghurt until you are happy with the spice level.

ROASTED TOMATO & MINT CHUTNEY

MAKES ABOUT 500ML (2 CUPS)

I do love a little olive oil in tomato chutneys like this. Olive oil is becoming increasingly popular in India, just like it is here. It isn't great for cooking curries, but with recipes like this, it's perfect!

PREP TIME: 5 MINS
COOKING TIME: 5 MINS

5 large Roma tomatoes
1 garlic clove, minced
Juice of 1 lime
1 tsp lime zest
½ tsp orange zest
2 green chillies
2 tbsp extra-virgin olive oil (optional)
2 tbsp roughly chopped coriander (cilantro)
3 tbsp roughly chopped mint
Salt, to taste

If you have a gas hob, place the tomatoes directly on the flame and blacken them all over. You can also do this under a hot grill in the oven. Either way, it will take about 5 minutes to blacken the tomatoes. Place the tomatoes in a food processor and add the remaining ingredients up to and including the mint. Blend to your liking, then season with salt.

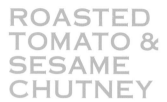

ROASTED TOMATO & SESAME CHUTNEY

MAKES ABOUT 500ML (2 CUPS)

This recipe was sent to me by my friend Santosh Shah, Executive Chef of Baluchi in London, to go with his chicken momos on page 20. What a delicious combo! I love this unique chutney and serve it with many other things too.

PREP TIME: 10 MINS
COOKING TIME: 10 MINS

4 large tomatoes
1 green chilli
100g (3½oz) sesame seeds
2 garlic cloves
5cm (2-inch) piece of ginger, peeled
50g (1¾oz) coriander (cilantro), roughly chopped
1 tsp mustard oil
Juice of ½ lemon
Salt, to taste

Char the whole tomatoes and chilli either over a gas flame or under a hot grill until blackened. This will take about 5 minutes. You can also do this on the barbecue. Remove the blackened skin if you like, but I usually leave it on. Set aside to cool.

Heat a frying pan over a medium heat and toast the sesame seeds until lightly browned and fragrant. Be sure to move the seeds around in the pan so that they toast evenly. Allow to cool.

Place all the ingredients up to and including the lemon juice in a food processor or blender and blend until you have a smooth chutney. Season with salt. This chutney can be served hot or cold.

LIGHT LIME PICKLE

MAKES ONE SMALL JAR (EASILY SERVES 4)

Although Indian pickles do often tend to have a lot of salt in them, it is important to point out that these pickles are used as a condiment as we in the West might use salt and pepper. Often, pickles are stirred into plain rice or served with bread, so the saltiness is not as strong as you might think. If adding a pickle like this to a meal, be sure to consider the salt when adding salt to other dishes. For example, don't add salt to the rice as you will get plenty of it from this pickle.

PREP TIME: 5 MINS
PLUS, PICKLING TIME

12 limes or more, if needed
4 tbsp salt
1 tsp ground turmeric
Chilli powder, to taste
1 level tsp ground fenugreek

Thoroughly wash and dry the limes. Cut six of them into very small pieces. If, like me, you prefer your lime pickles with larger chunks of lime, you could just quarter them. If using larger pieces, I recommend steaming them for about 15 minutes. If you're not sure, I suggest using finely chopped limes the first time you make this as it will appeal to more people and it's quicker to make. Place the lime pieces in a clean glass bowl and cut and squeeze the juice from the remaining limes over the top. The limes should be completely covered in the juice, so if they are not very juicy, you may need to squeeze a few more.

Stir in the remaining ingredients. For best results, refrigerate the pickle for at least one week before serving.

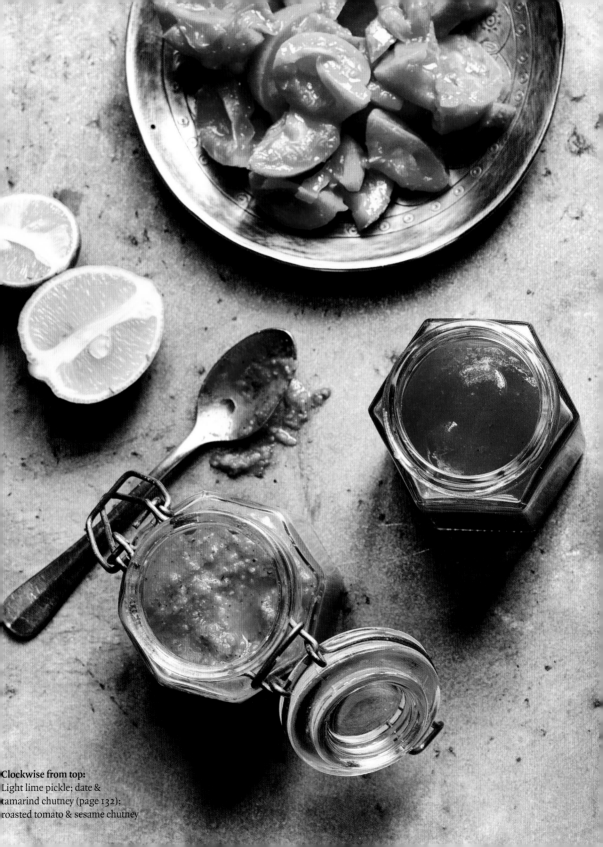

Clockwise from top:
Light lime pickle; date &
tamarind chutney (page 132);
roasted tomato & sesame chutney

10KCAL PER TBSP
2G CARBS PER TBSP

  7KCAL PER TBSP
0.7G CARBS PER TBSP

PICKLED PEAR ONIONS

MAKES ONE 500ML JAR (2 CUPS)

If you find it difficult to find pearl onions, another type of small onion or shallots can be used. I always try to source pearl onions, because I really like not only their flavour and texture, but also their appearance. The easiest way to peel pearl onions or shallots is to place them in a bowl and pour boiling hot water over them. Let stand for 30 seconds, then drain. Cover them with cold water so that they are cool enough to handle and drain again. The skins should come off easily. The beetroot in this recipe is there only to colour the pickle, so don't use it if you don't want to. You can use fresh or tinned (canned) beetroot for this one.

PREP TIME: 10 MINS
COOKING TIME: 5 MINS

20 pearl onions, peeled
125ml (½ cup) water
1 tsp finely chopped beetroot (optional)
2 cardamom pods, smashed
3 cloves
½ cinnamon stick
250ml (1 cup) white malt vinegar
2 tsp salt
1 tsp sugar or sugar substitute, to taste

Place the pearl onions in a sterilized jar. Heat the water in a saucepan until boiling, then add the beetroot, cardamom, cloves and cinnamon and let it all boil for about 2 minutes. Strain the water over the onions in the jar and stir in the vinegar and salt. Cover the jar and place it in the fridge. These will be ready after about 24 hours, but sometimes I sneak a few before that. Store in the fridge and use within two weeks. Personally, I prefer these unsweetened, but they are often sweetened with a little sugar or sugar substitute.

CUCUMBER RAITA

MAKES 300ML (1¼ CUPS)

I teach a tandoori cookery class regularly, and this cucumber raita is always served on the day. It goes so well with tandoori meats, seafood and vegetables, and is super easy to make too.

PREP TIME: 7 MINS

250g (1½ cups) low-fat Greek yoghurt
1 cucumber, peeled, seeded and grated
1 tbsp lemon juice
1 tbsp finely chopped mint or coriander (cilantro)
1 green chilli, finely chopped
Salt, to taste

Whisk the yoghurt until creamy smooth. Add the rest of the ingredients and stir well. That's it... job done. Check for seasoning and serve.

   6KCAL PER TBSP
0.7G CARBS PER TBSP

CORIANDER & CHILLI RAITA

MAKES 250ML (1 CUP)

This simple raita is the perfect accompaniment to the venison rogan josh on page 53. It's also delicious served with starters like onion bhajis and papadam cones. It is pictured on page 52.

PREP TIME: 5 MINS

100g (3½oz) coriander (cilantro)
2 green chillies
Juice of 1 lime
200g (7oz) fat-free yoghurt
Salt, to taste

Blend the coriander (cilantro), chillies and lime juice into a paste, then stir in the yoghurt and season with salt.

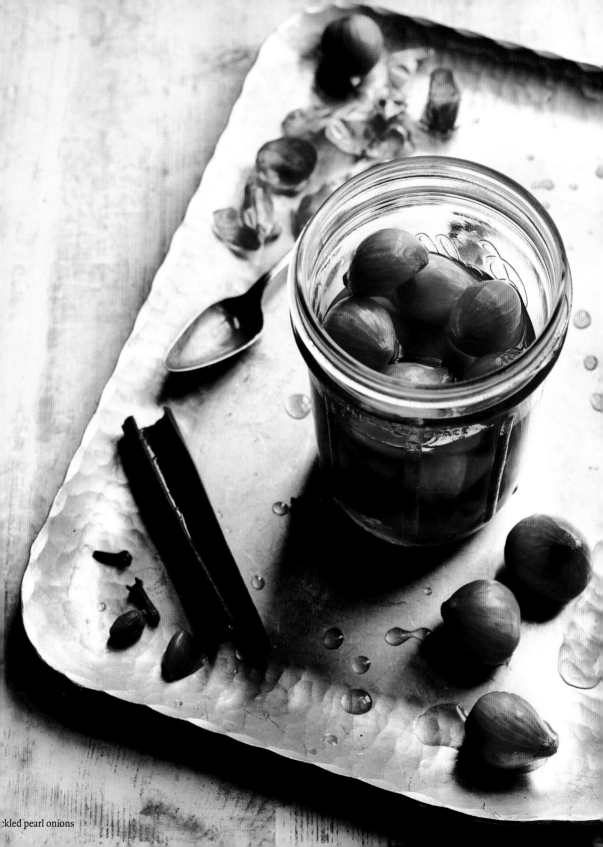

ckled pearl onions

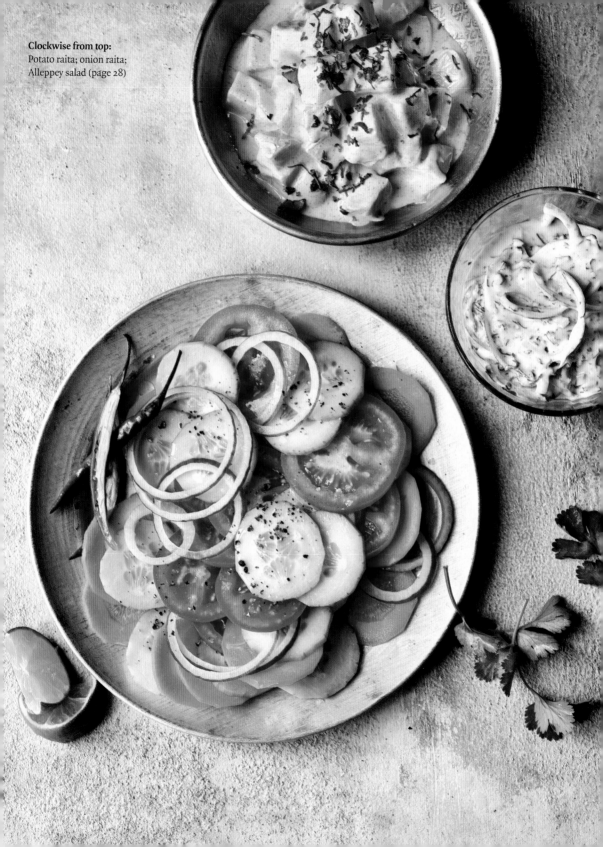

Clockwise from top:
Potato raita; onion raita;
Alleppey salad (page 28)

ONION RAITA

MAKES ABOUT 250ML (1 CUP)

POTATO RAITA

MAKES ABOUT 400ML (SCANT 1³/₄ CUPS)

Onion raita is good as a dip or served over biryani. One thing I like about making raitas is that my recipes change depending on what I feel like throwing in them at the time. A little garlic and ginger would be nice in this, for example. Never be afraid to experiment! If it sounds good, it probably will be.

PREP TIME: 5 MINS

175g (³/₄ cup) low-fat Greek yoghurt
½ tsp ground cumin
1 red or brown onion, halved, finely sliced and cut into
    2.5cm (1-inch) pieces
1 green chilli, finely chopped
2 tbsp finely chopped coriander (cilantro)
2 tbsp finely chopped mint leaves
About 60ml (¼ cup) water
Salt, to taste

In a large mixing bowl, whisk the yoghurt with the ground cumin. Add the remaining ingredients up to and including the mint leaves and whisk some more. Now gradually drizzle in the water to make a thinner raita until you are happy with the consistency. Season with salt and serve chilled.

I'm a big fan of raitas and usually like to serve a selection of them with a meal. Raitas offer a way of making a good meal awesome with all that added variety of flavour. Like most raitas, this keeps in the fridge well, so feel free to work ahead. You will see in the picture (at the top) that I cut the potatoes into fairly large but bite-sized chunks. If you prefer, you could cut them much smaller. This is delicious served over biryanis or as a dip.

PREP TIME: 10 MINS
COOKING TIME: 10–15 MINS

140g (5oz) potato (about 1 large or 2 medium), peeled
    and cut into small cubes
250g (1¼ cups) low-fat plain yoghurt
½ tsp ground cumin
½ tsp Kashmiri chilli powder (more or less to taste)
½ tsp chaat masala (see page 148)
2 tbsp finely chopped coriander (cilantro)
½ tsp mint sauce (optional)
Salt, to taste

Bring a pan of water to the boil and add the potato. Simmer for about 10 minutes, or until soft and cooked through. Drain and set aside to cool.

Meanwhile, place the yoghurt in a large mixing bowl. Add the cooled potatoes and the remaining ingredients and whisk well to combine.

MUSTARD & CORIANDER RAITA

MAKES ABOUT 250ML (1 CUP)

I like to serve this as a raita, but it also makes a delicious low-fat salad dressing. You can make a thinner dressing by stirring in a couple of tablespoons of fat-free milk.

PREP TIME: 5 MINS
COOKING TIME: 2 MINS

250g (1¼ cups) fat-free plain yoghurt
3 tbsp finely chopped coriander (cilantro)
1 tbsp honey
1 tbsp garlic and ginger paste
1 tbsp rapeseed (canola) oil
1 tsp mustard seeds
½ tsp ground turmeric
10 fresh or frozen curry leaves (optional)
Juice of 1 lime
Salt, to taste
2–3 tbsp fat-free milk (optional)

In a bowl, whisk the yoghurt until creamy smooth, then add the coriander, honey and ginger and garlic paste, and whisk to combine. Set aside.

Heat the oil in a small frying pan over a medium–high heat. Add the mustard seeds and temper them in the oil until they begin to pop (after about 30 seconds), then add the turmeric and curry leaves (if using) and fry for about 30 seconds until fragrant.

Pour the hot oil over the yoghurt mixture and whisk again so that the yoghurt doesn't curdle. Add the lime juice and season with salt. If using as a salad dressing, you might like to thin it with a little milk.

CREAMY AVOCADO RAITA

MAKES ABOUT 500ML (2 CUPS)

Believe me... this one is absolutely delicious served with homemade papadams! More often than not, I tend to use it as a creamy salad dressing or as a dip for crudités. If used as a salad dressing, a little goes a long way, so there's no need to drown your greens in it.

PREP TIME: 10 MINS

250g (1¼ cups) fat-free plain yoghurt
1 small bunch (about 15g/½oz) coriander (cilantro), chopped
Juice of 2 limes
1 garlic clove, smashed
2 fresh green chillies, chopped
½ tsp ground cumin
1 medium avocado, peeled, pitted and chopped
1 tbsp fat-free milk (optional)
Salt, to taste

Place the yoghurt, coriander, lime juice, garlic, green chillies, cumin and avocado in a blender and blend until smooth. For a thinner dressing, you can add a little milk. Stir in salt to taste.

NOTE

Looking for a flavour boost? Try adding a dash of red chilli sauce. If you like the idea, use your favourite brand. Just remember that most chilli sauces have plenty of salt in them, so add the sauce before adjusting the seasoning.

64KCAL
7.6G CARBS

SLICED RED ONION SALAD

SERVES 4 AS A GARNISH/SIDE SALAD

This is a real eye-catching salad that is used a lot as a garnish with grilled meats and seafood. You can see the finished salad on page 103.

PREP TIME: 25 MINS

2 red onions, thinly sliced
About ½ tsp salt
1–3 green chillies, finely chopped
2 medium tomatoes, deseeded and very finely sliced
125ml (½ cup) low-fat coconut milk
Juice of 1 lime (more or less, to taste)
Salt, to taste

Place the onions in a bowl with the salt. Let stand for about 20 minutes, then squeeze the water out of the onions and discard. Rinse the onions well and add the remaining ingredients to the onions and stir well to combine. Serve chilled as a garnish or side salad.

NOTE

Most of the calories in this salad are from the low-fat coconut milk. If you are really watching the calories, you can leave it out and the salad will still be delicious.

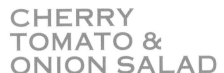

23KCAL
3.4G CARBS

CHERRY TOMATO & ONION SALAD

SERVES 4 AS A GARNISH/SIDE SALAD

If you're finding it difficult to source yellow cherry tomatoes, just use red ones, or try other varieties. I just like the appearance of this colourful combo.

PREP TIME: 10 MINS

1 small red onion, halved, finely sliced and cut into 2.5cm (1-inch) pieces
Juice of 2 limes
8 yellow cherry tomatoes, quartered
8 red cherry tomatoes, quartered
2 green chillies, thinly sliced
1 tsp olive oil (optional)
Salt and freshly ground black pepper, to taste

Place all the ingredients in a large salad bowl and mix well. Taste and season with salt and black pepper.

CARROT & COCONUT SALAD

SERVES 4 AS A GARNISH/SIDE SALAD

Although a small amount of sugar is usually added to this salad, I find the natural sweetness in the coconut and carrots to be enough for me, so I usually leave it out. You can see this finished and delicious salad next to the grilled seabass on page 119.

PREP TIME: 10 MINS
COOKING TIME: 10 MINS

100g (3½oz) fresh or frozen grated coconut
½ tsp rapeseed (canola) oil or cooking spray
10 cashew nuts, crushed
450g (1lb) grated carrots
Juice of 1 lime
½ tsp sugar or sugar substitute, to taste (optional)
Salt, to taste
½ tsp cumin seeds
3 green chillies, cut into thin rings

Heat a frying pan over a medium heat and toast the coconut until light brown. This only takes about 2 minutes, so watch it. Transfer to a large mixing bowl to cool.

Add the oil to the pan or spray it with cooking spray and toast the cashew nuts until light brown, stirring often so that they toast evenly. Place the cashews in a spice grinder or pestle and mortar and grind to a powder. Put the ground cashew nuts and carrots in the bowl with the coconut and add the lime juice, sugar (if using) and season with salt. Add the cumin seeds and green chillies to the pan and fry over a medium heat for about 30 seconds, or until the cumin is fragrant. Pour this mixture into the mixing bowl and stir well to combine. Check for seasoning and chill in the fridge before serving.

SPROUTED MOONG SALAD

SERVES 6

This salad is so good; I keep some on hand all the time. It keeps for days in the fridge and is a nice side for any meal.

PREP TIME: 10 MINS, PLUS SPROUTING TIME
COOKING TIME: 7 MINS

300g (2½ cups) sprouted moong lentils (see page 150)
1 tbsp rapeseed (canola) oil
½ tsp mustard seeds
1 dried red Kashmiri chilli
10 fresh or frozen curry leaves
½ tsp cumin seeds
¼ tsp ground turmeric
2 garlic cloves, minced
Juice of 1 lemon (about 1 tbsp)
1 tsp ground cumin
Salt and freshly ground black pepper, to taste
2 tomatoes, diced small
½ cucumber, diced small
1 green chilli, finely chopped
1 red onion, finely chopped
2 tbsp finely chopped coriander (cilantro), to garnish

Check the sprouted moong for any lentils that didn't sprout and remove them. Rinse the sprouts in a colander, then leave to drain.

Bring a saucepan of water to the boil and simmer the sprouts for about 5 minutes. Drain and set aside.

Heat the oil in a small saucepan over a medium–high heat. When hot, add the mustard seeds. When they begin to crackle (after about 30 seconds), add the dried red Kashmiri chillies and curry leaves. Reduce the heat to medium and stir in the cumin seeds and turmeric. After 1 minute, turn off the heat.

Pour this flavoured oil into a mixing bowl and whisk in the garlic, lemon juice and ground cumin. Taste and season with salt and black pepper. Add the sprouted moong, tomatoes, cucumber, chilli and onion. Toss well and check for seasoning again. Garnish with the coriander.

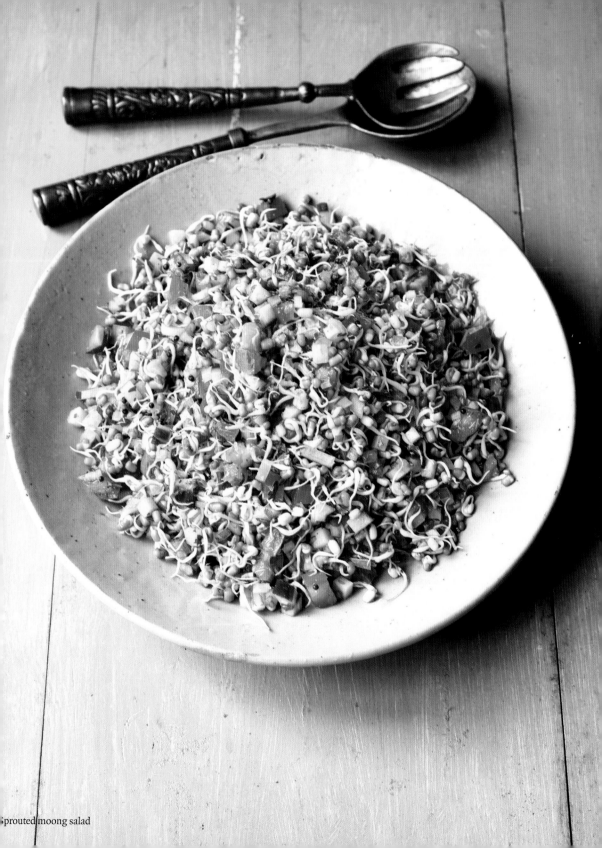

sprouted moong salad

BASICS

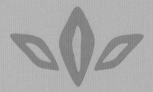

Here you'll find a selection of homemade spice blends and sauces that will take your curries up a notch. You can't beat the flavour and aroma that home-toasted and ground spices will add to your dishes. I have also revealed my no-fail method for sprouting lentils: all whole lentils can be sprouted at home. They are delicious added to sauces, used as a garnish or, as you can see on page 142, in a healthy salad. That's not all – you will also learn how to make no-fat caramelized onions and a low-sodium version with very little oil (page 151), both of which are delicious used in biryanis or stirred into sauces.

LAMB/CHICKEN STOCK SOUP
SERVES 4 AS A SOUP

This is a delicious and wholesome soup. Leave the coconut, chillies and chilli powder out and the same stock can be used to flavour curry-house-style curries (see pages 80–99). I often add a lot more cubed meat off the bone and then fish it out to use as pre-cooked meat in my curry-house-style curries. This recipe also works well as a vegetarian or vegan soup: leave the meat out and add more carrots and potatoes to your liking. You can also add other veggies like green beans, broccoli, aubergine (eggplant), chickpeas, kidney beans or whatever you think sounds good. When cooking this as a vegetable soup, just follow the recipe, but add chopped vegetables at the end and just cook them through so that they are not overcooked and mushy.

PREP TIME: 10 MINS
COOKING TIME: 30–90 MINS

2 tbsp (or less) rapeseed (canola) oil
6 green cardamom pods, smashed
7 cloves, lightly crushed
½ tsp cumin seeds
½ cinnamon stick
½ tsp black peppercorns
30 fresh or frozen curry leaves (optional)
2 medium onions, thinly sliced
3 green bird's eye chillies, cut into thin rings (optional)
5cm (2-inch) piece of ginger, peeled and finely chopped
6 garlic cloves, finely chopped
2 potatoes, cut into bite-sized chunks (optional)
1 large carrot, cut into thick rounds
750g (1lb 10oz) lamb or chicken on the bone
2 tomatoes, roughly chopped
1 tsp Kashmiri chilli powder
1 level tsp ground turmeric
400ml (1¾ cups) light coconut milk
Salt, to taste
1 tsp freshly ground black pepper (or to taste)
Chopped coriander (cilantro), to garnish (optional)

Heat the oil in a large saucepan over a medium–high heat. Stir in the cardamom pods, cloves, cumin seeds, cinnamon and black peppercorns and let these spices infuse in the oil for about 30 seconds. Stir in the curry leaves (if using) followed by the onions and fry over a medium heat for about 5 minutes until the onions are soft and translucent. Add the green chillies (if using), ginger and garlic, along with the potatoes (if using) and carrot and give it all a good stir to combine.

Add the meat and brown it for about 2 minutes, then stir in the tomatoes, chilli powder and ground turmeric. Add just enough water to cover (about 1 litre/4½ cups) and simmer until the meat is cooked through and tender. If using chicken, this should only take about 20 minutes; lamb can take 1 hour or more.

Add the coconut milk and simmer until you are happy with the consistency. Season with salt and black pepper. If you haven't used curry leaves, you could garnish with coriander for a little colour.

NOTE

This soup is also great for stock and pre-cooked meat and vegetables for curry-house curries.

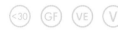

TOMATO PURÉE

This is simply a thin purée of tomatoes used in many curries for flavour and colour. Here are two ways you can make it.

1 tbsp concentrated tomato paste
3 tbsp water

Simply mix the ingredients together to form a thinner paste. This recipe can be easily scaled up or down: just use 1 part tomato paste to 3 parts water.

400g (14oz) canned (tinned) plum tomatoes
concentrated tomato paste, to taste (optional)

Blend the plum tomatoes to make a smooth purée. If you want a deeper red colour, add in a little concentrated tomato paste.

NOTE
You could also use sieved, unseasoned Italian passata.

GARAM MASALA
MAKES 3 GENEROUS TABLESPOONS

There are thousands, if not millions, of different recipes for garam masala. Garam masala is essentially just a selection of warming spices. In my past cookbooks, I gave my large batch recipe, which is great for convenience, but garam masala is best on the day you make it, so here I give you my small batch recipe. Feel free to scale it up and make a large batch to have on hand. It will keep well stored in an airtight container for up to three months without much loss of flavour. That amazing aroma you get on the day you toast and grind it only lasts for about a day though.

PREP TIME: 5 MINS
COOKING TIME: 1 MIN

1 tbsp cumin seeds
1 tbsp coriander seeds
¾ tbsp fennel seeds
¼ cinnamon stick
3 cloves
Seeds from 6 green cardamom
    pods
1 tsp black peppercorns
1.5cm (¾-inch) piece of mace

Heat a small dry frying pan over a medium–high heat and add all the spices. Move the spices around in the pan so that they toast evenly, until they become fragrant and warm to the touch. If they begin to smoke, you have burnt them and they will become bitter.

Remove the spices from the heat, transfer to a plate to cool, then grind to a fine powder in a spice grinder or pestle and mortar.

RECHEADO MASALA
MAKES 500ML (2 CUPS)

Recheado masala is used a lot in Goan cooking. There are many different recipes, but they are all quite similar. Goan food was heavily influenced by the Portuguese and 'recheado' means 'stuffed' in Portuguese. So the name isn't, as many think, describing what is in the masala, but the fact that it is stuffed into fish, vegetables and meat before cooking. In this recipe, I suggest using tequila, which tastes very much like Goan coconut and cashew feni, a triple-distilled alcohol that is used a lot in Goan cooking but is not available for purchase outside of Goa. You can, of course, scale this recipe up or down depending on how much you need, but it does keep very well in the fridge for at least three months and probably much longer.

PREP TIME: 15 MINS
COOKING TIME: 3 MINS

20 dried Kashmiri chillies
1 tsp cumin seeds
½ tbsp black peppercorns
½ tsp black mustard seeds
4 cloves
½ cinnamon stick
6 fenugreek seeds
2 tbsp garlic and ginger paste
1–3 green bird's eye chillies,
    roughly chopped
1 tsp ground turmeric
1 tsp tamarind paste (see page
    149) or concentrate
1 tsp jaggery or sugar
250ml (1 cup) white wine vinegar
    or coconut vinegar
250ml (1 cup) tequila, or more
    vinegar
Salt, to taste

Heat a dry frying pan over a medium–high heat and toast the dried chillies, cumin seeds, black peppercorns, mustard seeds, cloves, cinnamon and fenugreek seeds for 2 minutes. Stir regularly so that the spices toast evenly. When fragrant and warm to the touch, remove the spices from the heat and transfer to a plate to cool. Place the spices in a spice grinder and grind to a fine powder. Add the remaining ingredients up to and including the tequila and blend to a smooth paste. Season with salt and store in an airtight jar in the fridge until required.

TANDOORI MASALA
MAKES 5 TABLESPOONS

My tandoori masala is a lot more complex than most commercially available brands. Most shop-bought tandoori masalas are a combination of cumin, coriander, salt and citric acid powder. They work well, but I hope you give this one a try. This is a small batch, so feel free to scale it up if you want to make more. It will keep in an airtight container in a dry location for a good couple of months without much loss of flavour.

PREP TIME: 3 MINS
COOKING TIME: 3 MINS

1 tbsp coriander seeds
1 tbsp cumin seeds
1 tsp black mustard seeds
½ cinnamon stick, broken into pieces
1 small piece of mace
1 tsp ground ginger
2 tsp garlic powder
2 tsp dried onion powder
2 tsp amchoor (dried mango powder)
1 tsp red food colour powder (optional)

Heat a dry frying pan over a medium–high heat and add the coriander seeds, cumin seeds, black mustard seeds, cinnamon and mace. Toast, moving the spices around in the pan, until they are fragrant and warm to the touch but not smoking.

Transfer to a plate to cool slightly. Place in a spice grinder or pestle and mortar and grind to a fine powder. Add the remaining ingredients and blend well. This spice blend will keep for up to two months in an airtight container with little loss of flavour, but is best used on the day you make it.

CHAAT MASALA
MAKES ABOUT 4 TABLESPOONS

If I know I'm going to be using a lot of chaat masala, I double or triple the quantities. Usually, chaat masala is used in small amounts, so I tend to make it in small batches. I love the flavour of the black salt, but it's one of those flavours that isn't at the top of everyone's list. Give this a try though.

PREP TIME: 5 MINS
COOKING TIME: 2 MINS

1 tbsp coriander seeds
1 tbsp cumin seeds
2 tsp amchoor (dried mango powder)
1 tsp garam masala (see page 146)
1 tbsp ground black salt
1 tsp freshly ground black pepper

Heat a dry frying pan over a medium–high heat and add the coriander seeds and cumin seeds. Toast, moving the spices around in the pan, until they are fragrant and warm to the touch but not smoking.

Transfer to a plate to cool slightly. Place in a spice grinder or pestle and mortar and grind to a fine powder. Add the remaining ingredients and blend well. This spice blend will keep for up to two months in an airtight container with little loss of flavour, but is best used on the day you make it.

TAMARIND PASTE

MAKES 500ML (2 CUPS)

Tamarind concentrate can be purchased in jars, but homemade tamarind paste is so much better. The paste can be stirred into curries as a souring agent. I use it in many of the recipes in this book. It can be made thicker, or you could add more water for a thinner paste or tamarind water.

PREP TIME: 40 MINS

200g (7oz) block of tamarind
400ml (1¾ cups) boiling water

Break the tamarind block into small pieces into a mixing bowl. Pour the boiling water over it and let it stand for 30 minutes. You could use a spoon to break up the tamarind into smaller pieces. After 30 minutes, use your hands to break up the tamarind even more, then pass through a fine-mesh sieve into another bowl. Any seeds that are left behind should be discarded. It will keep for months in a sterilized airtight glass jar in the fridge. I find this recipe perfect for my tastes, but you could simmer the paste for a few minutes to make it more concentrated.

BAFAT CURRY POWDER

MAKES ENOUGH FOR TWO CURRIES TO SERVE 4

Bafat curry powder is a really hot spice blend enjoyed mostly by the Christian population in Goa. It's a key ingredient for the pork bafat recipe on page 48, but it is also good stirred into so many things, as you would any spicy curry powder. Add it sparingly to stir-fried vegetables or other curry sauces. As you can see from the recipe, this is meant to give a dish a spicy boost, so I recommend toasting and grinding the spices on the day you are serving the dish you are making. This recipe doesn't produce much, but you can easily scale it up if you want to have some on hand all the time. If you like, you could also omit or reduce the amount of red chillies for a milder curry powder.

PREP TIME: 5 MINS
COOKING TIME: 5 MINS

30 dried Kashmiri chillies
1 cinnamon stick
2 tsp black peppercorns
2 tbsp cumin seeds
4 tbsp coriander seeds
2 star anise
4 cloves
1 tsp black mustard seeds
½ tsp ground turmeric

Heat a dry frying pan over a medium–high heat and add all the ingredients, except the turmeric. Toast, moving the spices around in the pan, until they are fragrant and warm to the touch but not smoking.

Transfer to a plate to cool slightly. Place the spices, including the turmeric, in a spice grinder or pestle and mortar and grind to a fine powder. This spice blend will keep for up to two months in an airtight container with little loss of flavour, but is best used on the day you make it.

MIXED POWDER

MAKES 17 TABLESPOONS

This is a special curry powder that is used a lot in UK curry houses. Although recipes do vary slightly from chef to chef, this version is one that I know works. It will give you that curry-house curry flavour you're looking for. Although you could simply use a good-quality shop-bought curry powder when mixed powder is call for in a recipe, this is simply better, especially if you make your own garam masala and curry powder to go in it. The madras curry powder in my book *The Curry Guy* and the bafat curry powder in this book (see page 149) both work well in this recipe.

PREP TIME: 2 MINS

1 tbsp garam masala (see page 146)
4 tbsp curry powder
3 tbsp ground turmeric
3 tbsp paprika
3 tbsp ground cumin
3 tbsp ground coriander

Mix all the spices together in a bowl and use as required. If you would like to make more or less, simply substitute tablespoons for teaspoons. I have a really good curry powder recipe in my first cookbook, *The Curry Guy*, but if you don't have it, any good-quality curry powder could be used.

SPROUT YOUR OWN LENTILS

PRODUCES SPROUTS THAT COME CLOSE TO FILLING A 2-LITRE BOTTLE

Any dried, whole lentils and pulses can be sprouted. These make fantastic-looking and edible garnishes. Here you will sprout moong lentils, which can be used in the sprouted moong lentil salad on page 142.

PREP TIME: 6 DAYS

200g (1 cup) whole green moong lentils

Day 1: Rinse the lentils under cold running water and place in a 2-litre plastic drinks bottle. Almost fill the bottle with fresh water and soak overnight.

Day 2: Make about 20 small holes in the bottle above the lentil line using a sharp knife. This will allow air in and also make it easier to drain the water. Pour the water out, then place the bottle in a warm location, but out of direct sunlight.

Days 3–4: Pour more fresh water over the lentils in the bottle and drain again. Do this for the next few days and watch those sprouts grow.

Days 5–6: When the lentils have sprouted, cut off the top of the bottle so that the sprouts can be easily removed. Store them in a clean bowl in the fridge, covered with cling film. They will keep that way for about one week.

CARAMELIZED ONIONS – TWO WAYS

MAKES ENOUGH FOR 1 CURRY TO SERVE 4

One of the drawbacks about trying to fry with less oil is that it takes longer. With onions playing such a big part in curries, I wanted to include the following two recipes that could come in handy and save you time. The caramelized onions can be kept in the fridge in an airtight container for up to four days or frozen for up to three months. These recipes can easily be scaled up and used as a base for your favourite dishes that call for fried onions. You could also blend the caramelized onions into a paste to use to thicken and add flavour to sauces or mix into seekh kebab meat. Stir them into a good raita. Just use your imagination... caramelized onions are delicious in so many things.

PREP TIME: 5 MINS
COOKING TIME: 20–25 MINS

NO-FAT CARAMELIZED ONIONS

2 onions
1 generous teaspoon fine salt

Thinly slice or finely chop the onions and sprinkle with the salt. Heat a non-stick frying pan over a medium heat and add the salted onions. Fry for 20–25 minutes, stirring continuously, until the onions turn deep brown in colour. If it looks like the onions are burning, reduce the heat a little and add a drop of water – not too much though. You want to caramelize the onions, not boil them!

LOW-SODIUM CARAMELIZED ONIONS

2 onions
A pinch of salt (optional)
2 teaspoons rapeseed (canola) oil

Thinly slice or finely chop the onions and sprinkle lightly with salt (if using). The salt helps release moisture from the onions so that they caramelize quicker, but you can caramelize them without salt.

Heat the oil in a frying pan over a medium heat. Fry the onions for 20–25 minutes, stirring continuously, until the onions turn deep brown in colour. If it looks like the onions are burning, add a drop of water – but not too much. If you add too much water, the onions will boil rather than caramelize.

INGREDIENTS

AJWAIN (CAROM) SEEDS

Ajwain 'seeds' are not actually seeds but small pieces of fruit. They smell a lot like thyme, though their flavour is more like a cross between oregano and fennel seeds but much stronger. They have a pungent, bitter flavour that can quickly overpower a dish, so should be used sparingly.

AMCHOOR (DRIED MANGO POWDER)

Amchoor powder has a tangy flavour that is used in many recipes to give them a delicious citric flavour. It is made by grinding dried mangos into a fine powder. If you can't find it, simply add a squeeze of lime or lemon juice to the finished dish. It is available from Asian shops, online and many supermarkets.

ASAFOETIDA

In its raw powder form, asafoetida smells a bit strange. Once fried, its aroma and flavour are much more pleasing – like fried onions. This spice is used sparingly as it is quite strong. In India, it is used as a substitute for garlic and onions in areas where consuming these is forbidden for religious reasons. Asafoetida is also an anti-flatulent and is cooked into dhals and bean dishes to ease digestion. Raw asafoetida is a key ingredient in chaat masala (see below), so it doesn't have to be cooked. Please note that some brands contain wheat flour, so if you are gluten-free, check the packaging.

BASMATI RICE

White basmati rice is served at Indian restaurants everywhere. It has a nutty flavour that is all its own. White basmati rice benefits from ageing, so look for the longest grain and longest aged basmati you can find. In my opinion, white basmati rice is one of the best, second only to the much healthier matta rice (see page 154). White basmati, like all white rice, has been processed and stripped of the outer pericarp and therefore most of its health benefits. About a year ago, I started using brown basmati, which is the same rice but unprocessed, and although I still prefer white, it is very good. It does take longer to cook, however. Strangely, my family prefer the much nuttier flavour and texture of brown basmati, so I recommend giving it a try.

BLACK MUSTARD SEEDS

Black (and brown) mustard seeds are hugely popular in Indian cooking. Although often toasted and used in different ground spice blends, they are most often tempered into hot oil over a high heat to release their pungent flavour. Most spices require a much lower temperature so that they don't burn and become bitter, but mustard seeds need the higher heat so that they crackle and release their flavour. For this reason, you will notice that they are usually added to the pan first over a high heat, then the heat is reduced before adding the other spices.

CHAAT MASALA

Like garam masala (see page 153) and curry powder, chaat masala is a popular spice blend that is often sprinkled over savoury and sweet chaats and even fruit. There are numerous recipes for it that normally include spices like cumin and coriander, but its key ingredients – those that make it stand out from the others – are black salt, asafoetida, amchoor (dried mango powder) and often chilli powder. The black salt gives it a sulphuric flavour and aroma that can take some getting used to, but try it a few times and you'll probably be hooked on it, like me. My recipe is on page 148.

COCONUT (GRATED)

Many of the recipes in this book call for fresh or frozen grated coconut. I usually crack open a coconut and grate it. Once you remove the hard brown shell, everything else is edible, even the thin brown skin. A very close 'second best' is frozen grated coconut, which I prefer to dried. This is available from almost all Asian shops. If using dried grated coconut, soak it in water for about an hour before using to rehydrate it, then strain out the excess water.

COCONUT AMINO

Coconut amino is an excellent, gluten-free alternative to soy sauce. It is very popular in Indian cooking and I actually prefer it to soy sauce. It is now available in many supermarkets, Asian shops and online.

COCONUT MILK

You will notice that the recipes in this book call for light coconut milk. Coconut milk is made by grating fresh coconut and adding a little water. The grated coconut is then squeezed to extract a thick, creamy milk, which is what you get when you purchase full-fat coconut milk. The process is then repeated to make light coconut milk. There simply wasn't room in this book to go into this process in detail, but luckily you can purchase great-quality tinned (canned) full-fat and light coconut milk in every supermarket. I find that light coconut milk works exceptionally well with these recipes, but if you aren't counting calories, you can use full-fat coconut milk too.

COCONUT OIL

Many nutritionists say that coconut oil is good for you; many others say it's not. I'll let you research and decide for yourself, but it is used a lot in south-Indian cooking and when used sparingly, as it is in this book, it probably won't do much harm. It is available from Asian shops and most supermarkets. When you purchase it, it is solid white but melts when it hits the hot pan. It doesn't really have a strong flavour of coconut, so other healthier oils like rapeseed (canola) oil can be substituted without much loss of flavour.

CURRY LEAVES

Fresh curry leaves are one of my favourite ingredients. You can find them in Asian shops, online and also in some supermarkets. If you purchase fresh curry leaves they can be frozen for future use, but use them within three months. Personally, I find dried curry leaves flavourless and a waste of money. By the way, when my recipes call for a certain number of curry leaves, don't take it too seriously. I often throw a big handful of the healthy leaves into a sauce at the end of cooking just because I like them so much.

FINE SEV

Sev comes in fine and also thicker forms. It is a fried noodle-like product made from gram flour. Fine sev is similar in appearance to angel hair pasta and is a popular topping for many chaats. It is available online and from many Asian shops. If you can't find it, you could substitute thicker varieties or just leave it out. I love the crunchiness it adds to chaats and how it improves presentation, making the dish much more interesting in appearance.

GARAM MASALA

This is a mixture of warming spices such as cinnamon, cumin, coriander seeds, cardamom seeds, mace and black peppercorns. You can purchase bags of whole spice garam masala from Asian shops, but I usually purchase the whole spices individually and come up with my own blends. These can be tempered into hot oil whole, but for the recipes in this book, the garam masala you need is ground, which is also available online, from Asian shops and many supermarkets. For best results, however, you should roast and grind your own. My recipe is on page 147.

GRAM (CHICKPEA) FLOUR

Gram flour is used all over India and is especially popular in pakoras. It is gluten free and is available from Asian shops and most supermarkets.

KOKUM

In all my years of cooking Indian food, there are a handful of ingredients that just blow me away because of their amazing and unique flavours. Kokum is one of them. Used mainly in south-Indian cooking, kokum is the dried rind of the kokum berry. The rinds are dried and used as a souring agent in sauces, just like tamarind is used in so many Indian dishes. I love it for its slightly smoky and sour flavour. The kokum rinds are not supposed to be eaten because they are so sour, though before I knew that I ate a few and actually quite liked them! Kokum can be hard to come by outside India, but it is available online, so please take the time to order and try it in the recipes that call for it. As I mention in the recipes, you can substitute other souring agents like tamarind or lemon/lime juice, but in those recipes calling for kokum, there is a delicious and even eye-opening reason for it.

LENTILS

In this book there are recipes that call for chana dhal, white split urad dhal and toor dhal (aka split pigeon pea) lentils. All of these are widely available from Asian grocers and online. Many supermarkets stock them now too.

MATTA RICE

Also known as rosematta rice, Kerala red rice and Goan red rice, matta rice is a parboiled rice that is loved for its earthy, rich flavour. It is also a lot better for you than white rice as the red pericarp is left on it, just as the pericarp is left on brown rice. That said, I find it so much more enjoyable to eat than brown rice as its flavour and texture go well with any curry, or simply eaten with pickles and chutneys. As the pericarp has not been removed, it is a healthy choice, containing loads of vitamins, unlike white rice, which has been processed. I still love white basmati rice, but now actually prefer matta rice. It is available online and from many Asian shops. My recipe for aromatic matta rice is on page 123.

MIXED POWDER

Mixed powder is essentially a curry powder and is easy to make using store-bought ground spices. It is one of the secret ingredients in making BIR (British Indian Restaurant)-style curries. You will find my homemade mixed powder recipe on page 150, but if time is an issue, you could substitute a good-quality shop-bought curry powder.

MUSTARD OIL

There is no substitute for mustard oil, and I love the stuff! It has a pungent and strong flavour and has been used for centuries in northern India and Bangladeshi cooking. It is available in the UK but has not been approved for human consumption, probably because no one has bothered to try to get it approved. You'll find it in the hair aisle at Asian shops. If you decide to break the rules as I often do, be sure to heat it up until it reaches smoking point, then let it cool before using. This purifies it. Sometimes when I'm feeling lazy, I skip that step though, especially when so little is required in most recipes.

NIGELLA SEEDS (BLACK ONION SEEDS)

Although nigella seeds are often called black onion seeds, they aren't actually from the onion family. Whatever you call them, they are excellent sprinkled over homemade naans. If you are not familiar with them by name, you will almost definitely recognize their flavour and aroma when used.

PANEER

This is the most simple of cheeses. Indian paneer is now widely available from Asian shops and in supermarkets. For the recipes in this book, commercially bought paneer will do fine, but you can make your own too. I have a recipe for homemade paneer on my website www.greatcurryrecipes.net and also in my book *The Curry Guy Veggie*.

RICE FLOUR

Rice flour is gluten free and is the perfect alternative for cornflour (cornstarch). Often, the two different flours are used in one recipe, but you could substitute more rice flour or cornflour if you want to go gluten free.

TAMARIND

Tamarind is a souring agent that is used a lot in Indian cooking. It is available in both block form from Asian shops and as a concentrate that is available almost everywhere now. The concentrate is quite strong and should be added to taste until you are happy with the sourness of the dish. I prefer the flavour of homemade tamarind paste (concentrate), which is made from block tamarind. If you've got the will and the time, try my recipe on page 149. If you find tamarind difficult to source or you just don't have it on hand, try adding a little lemon or lime juice to get a nice sour and tart flavour. The juice won't be the same, but it is a good substitute that will work.

TURMERIC (GROUND)

Known for its woody and earthy flavour, turmeric is a super spice that is hugely popular in Indian food, not only for its flavour but also its yellow colour. There are so many health benefits in turmeric! Studies have shown that it can prevent and even treat cancer, it is an anti-inflammatory, reduces the risk of heart disease and can even increase brain function and reduce the risk of brain diseases. I could go on, but this is a cookbook not a medical book. Use sparingly as it can quickly overpower a dish, and enjoy!

SUPPLIERS & CLASSES

INGREDIENTS

SPICE KITCHEN ONLINE LTD

Spice Kitchen supplies excellent quality spices that can be purchased online. Not only that, it has begun producing the spice blends from my books, such as mixed powder, curry powder, garam masala, tandoori masala and chaat masala. It also supplies kokum, which is called for in many of my recipes. You can order spice tins/masala dabbas filled with whole spices or its own spice blends from around the world, which are all blended in-house.

www.spicekitchenuk.com; 07729 116102 soldwithlove@spicekitchenuk.com

EAST END FOODS

East End Foods has been a much valued sponsor of my blog for many years. I have visited their production facilities and can trust them to deliver excellent quality spices, pulses, flours and rice. Their whole and ground spices are available at supermarkets, Asian grocers and from online retailers all over the UK.

https://eastendfoods.co.uk

SPICES OF INDIA

In addition to all the groceries and spices they supply, you will also find a fantastic range of Indian kitchen and tableware.

www.spicesofindia.co.uk

PLANTS4PRESENTS

This company supplies plants, such as curry leaf plants and different chilli plants, which you can have delivered to your home.

www.plants4presents.co.uk

BALTI BOWLS

THE BIRMINGHAM BALTI BOWL CO.

Here you can purchase authentic steel-pressed Balti bowls, manufactured in Birmingham. They come stylishly presented in a gift box.

www.thebirminghambaltibowlco.com

BARBECUE & GRILLING

THÜROS BARBECUES

If you love kebabs, you've got to check out Thüros Kebab Grills. I love mine.

www.thueros.com

TRAEGER BARBECUES

The easy way to get delicious smoky flavour into your barbecued foods. Traeger barbecues use wood pellets to cook the food. You can set the preferred temperature and the let the Traeger do all the work. This is the perfect barbecue for easy indirect cooking.

www.thealfrescochef.co.uk/find-a-dealer

COOKING CLASSES

BIG IN FRANCE

Big in France specializes in cooking holidays at their beautiful villa in Vendée, France. I teach annual weekend-long curry classes there.

www.biginfrance.com

MY UK CURRY CLASSES

I teach cooking classes around the UK. For more information, please visit my website.

www.greatcurryrecipes.net

US SOURCES

PENZEYS

Large range spices that can be purchased online.

www.penzeys.com

SAVORY SPICE

Large range of spices.

www.savoryspiceshop.com

ISHOPINDIAN.COM

Groceries and Indian cooking utensils.

www.ishopindian.com

ANCIENT COOKWARE

A large range of cookware from India and around the world.

www.ancientcookware.com

INDEX

ACKNOWLEDGEMENTS

It was a pleasure to work with Quadrille again to produce this book. I would like to thank Sarah Lavelle for commissioning the project and my editor Louise Francis for helping bring the book together. I am also grateful to copy-editor Corinne Masciocchi for her work in the early stages and dietitian Sian Porter for ensuring the recipes ticked the boxes for a light cookbook.

Great photography makes a cookbook and it has been fun working with photographer Kris Kirkham again. I love how he brings my recipes to life through his photography. I would also like to thank food stylist Tamara Vos for her artistic way of making the recipes look amazing.

Since I started my blog, I have tried to meet and learn from the best chefs. Thank you to Jomon Kuriakose, the Chef de Cuisine at Baluchi in LaLit London, who went out of his way to show me some of the best eateries in Kochi, Kerala, and to Santosh Shah, Executive Chef at Baluchi, who also gave me recipes.

I am grateful to Chef Shihabudeen VM, who made us the most amazing breakfast ever at his family home near Kochi and has been very open with his recipes and advice, and to Chef Vipin VU in Alleppey, who lent me his family cookbook.

Thank you to chef Moh Hoque for teaching me the chicken wing recipe on page 24 while I was teaching a tandoori class with him. Thank you to Nick Jones for your tandoor instruction and for supplying me with my own home Tandoor-i, which I use daily to develop recipes.

I would also like to thank Rahul Krishnan Muttumpuram, Executive Chef at Cheenavala Seafood Restaurant in Kochi. Your recipes and food are top notch. There's no way I could leave out Aneesh Prasad from the Crown Plaza for inviting us to Trilogy in the Crown Plaza, Kochi where I met Chef Rejimon and Chef Anand. Their food was awesome and I can't wait to return. Thank you also to my literary agent Clare Hulton for once again making this all happen.

Lastly, thank you for purchasing this cookbook. I hope you enjoy the recipes.

Publishing Director: Sarah Lavelle
Project Editor: Louise Francis
Consultant Dietitian: Sian Porter
Senior Designer: Nicola Ellis
Junior Designer: Alicia House
Cover Design: Smith & Gilmour
Photographer: Kris Kirkham
Food Stylist: Tamara Vos
Food Stylist Assistants:
Lucinda Notley, Olivia Williamson
Props Stylist: Faye Wears
Head of Production: Stephen Lang
Production Controller: Sinead Hering

First published in 2020 by Quadrille,
an imprint of Hardie Grant Publishing

Quadrille
52–54 Southwark Street,
London SE1 1UN
www.quadrille.com

Text © 2020 Dan Toombs
Photography © 2020 Kris Kirkham
Design and layout © 2020 Quadrille Publishing Ltd

Cataloguing-in-Publication Data. A catalogue record for this book is available from the British Library.

ISBN 978-1-78713-461-4

Reprinted in 2020
10 9 8 7 6 5 4 3 2

Printed in China

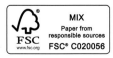

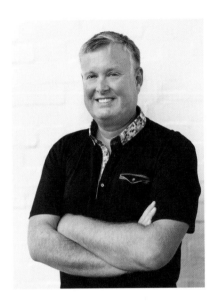

In five short years Dan took The Curry Guy from an idea to a reliable brand. The recipes are all developed and tested in Dan's home kitchen. And they work. His bestselling first cookbook – *The Curry Guy* – and the 130,000 curry fans who visit his blog every month can testify to that fact.

www.greatcurryrecipes.net | @thecurryguy